AF887593

Physeo

TABLE OF CONTENTS

We would like to extend a special thanks to the following individuals who have spent countless hours and support to make Physeo possible.

Ajay Davidson, MD

Alexandra Galel, MD

Alexandra Harding

Anissa Laine Bayabos Amilhamja

Anne-Sophie van Wingerden
Medical Student
Columbia Vagelos College of Physicians and Surgeons

Antonio Acevedo

Ayan Agarwal
MBBS Student
Vardhman Mahavir Medical College and Safdarjung Hospital
New Delhi, India

Brianna Cocuzzo, MsC

Brooke Walsh, MS

Camelita Thrift

Christopher A. Price, MS

Genevieve Saliuk
MD Candidate 2024
UTMB School of Medicine

George Myo Win, BS
University of Missouri-Columbia School of Medicine

Ghadeer Magdy Elshafey, MD

H. Robert Cannon, DO

Dr. Jabran Wasti, House Officer
Dr. Ruth K.M. Pfau Civil Hospital
Karachi, Pakistan

Jae Cheol Bae

Dr. James Nunn

Jennifer M. Locke, BA
MD Candidate

Justin Wong, DO

Kurestin Miller, BA
MD Candidate

Lauren S. Faber, MD

Lauren Schwartz

Lee Azolai

Leslie Jewett, MD

Logan B. Carlyle, OMS-II

Marisol Cárdenas Calderón, MD

Mark Parry, MD, Resident Physician
Department of Obstetrics and Gynecology
OhioHealth – Riverside Methodist
Columbus, Ohio

Mason T. Bennet

Mateo Betancourt Escobar
Universidad Autónoma de San Luis
Potosí, Mexico

Mohamed Elshennawy

Natalia Kerr, MD

Nijat Aliyev, MD

Nikoloz Karazanashvili

Nirupamaa Sivanushanthan
Medical Student

Ostapenko Karolina

Dr. Rahil Patel, Medical Officer
Sharda Hospital
New Delhi, India

Mr. Rishabh Goyal

Roaa Zayat, MD

Rojin Arefi, MD

Ryan Zia

We would like to extend a special thanks to the following individuals who have spent countless hours and support to make Physeo possible.

Ajay Davidson, MD

Alexandra Galel, MD

Alexandra Harding

Anissa Laine Bayabos Amilhamja

Anne-Sophie van Wingerden
Medical Student
Columbia Vagelos College of Physicians and Surgeons

Antonio Acevedo

Ayan Agarwal
MBBS Student
Vardhman Mahavir Medical College and Safdarjung Hospital
New Delhi, India

Brianna Cocuzzo, MsC

Brooke Walsh, MS

Camelita Thrift

Christopher A. Price, MS

Genevieve Saliuk
MD Candidate 2024
UTMB School of Medicine

George Myo Win, BS
University of Missouri-Columbia School of Medicine

Ghadeer Magdy Elshafey, MD

H. Robert Cannon, DO

Dr. Jabran Wasti, House Officer
Dr. Ruth K.M. Pfau Civil Hospital
Karachi, Pakistan

Jae Cheol Bae

Dr. James Nunn

Jennifer M. Locke, BA
MD Candidate

Justin Wong, DO

Kurestin Miller, BA
MD Candidate

Lauren S. Faber, MD

Lauren Schwartz

Lee Azolai

Leslie Jewett, MD

Logan B. Carlyle, OMS-II

Marisol Cárdenas Calderón, MD

Mark Parry, MD, Resident Physician
Department of Obstetrics and Gynecology
OhioHealth – Riverside Methodist
Columbus, Ohio

Mason T. Bennet

Mateo Betancourt Escobar
Universidad Autónoma de San Luis
Potosí, Mexico

Mohamed Elshennawy

Natalia Kerr, MD

Nijat Aliyev, MD

Nikoloz Karazanashvili

Nirupamaa Sivanushanthan
Medical Student

Ostapenko Karolina

Dr. Rahil Patel, Medical Officer
Sharda Hospital
New Delhi, India

Mr. Rishabh Goyal

Roaa Zayat, MD

Rojin Arefi, MD

Ryan Zia

Salikh Murtaliev, MD

Sarah Jaber, D.O.
Internal Medicine Physician

Sergio R. Ortiz, MD, MPH

Shawna-Kay Young
MD Student

Shelia Chandrahas

Soomal Zukhruf Memon

Sumit Raut

Syed Ali Haider

Syed Awais Ahmed, MD

Tori Walsh

Tamari Papidze

Telyn Peterson, OMS-III
Rocky Vista University
Southern Utah

Trey Edwards, DO

Warda Hameed, MD

Yasmeen Abdulrahman, MD

Yomna Dean, MS-4

Zurabi Zaalishvili, MD

Emergency Medicine | Section 1: Abdominal Trauma

I. Blunt Abdominal Trauma: Definition
  A. Physical trauma
    1. Physical attack
    2. High-velocity impact
    3. Damage to internal organs

II. Blunt Abdominal Trauma: Pathophysiology
  A. Shearing (e.g. distal aortic rupture, hepatic tear)
  B. Crushing (most commonly affecting spleen, liver, kidney)
  C. Compression (e.g. bursting or rupture of vessels)
  D. Hollow organ rupture (e.g. stomach, intestines, gallbladder) → infection
  E. Solid-organ injury (e.g. liver, spleen, pancreas) → hypovolemia

III. Blunt Abdominal Trauma: Etiologies
  A. Vehicle accident (e.g. seat belt injury)
  B. Falls
  C. Industrial and recreational accidents
  D. Iatrogenic (e.g. cardiac resuscitation, Heimlich maneuver)
  E. Sports injury

IV. Blunt Abdominal Trauma: Clinical Features
  A. Nausea, vomiting
  B. Abdominal pain, tenderness
  C. Diminished or absent bowel sounds
  D. Abdominal distention and rigidity
  E. Pneumoperitoneum
  F. Physical exam findings (e.g. abrasions, contusions, lacerations, bone fractures)

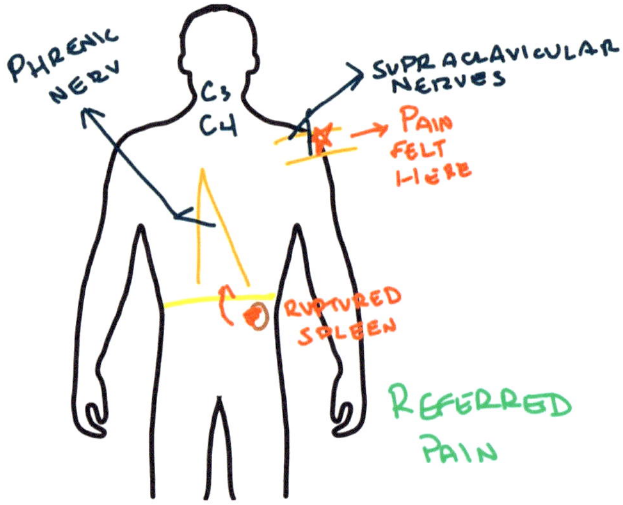

FIGURE 14.1.1 - Kehr Sign in Splenic Rupture

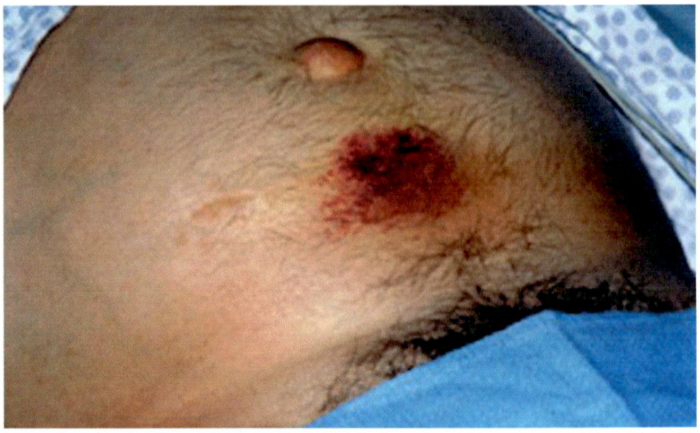

FIGURE 14.1.2 - Cullen Sign Suggesting Intraperitoneal Hemorrhage

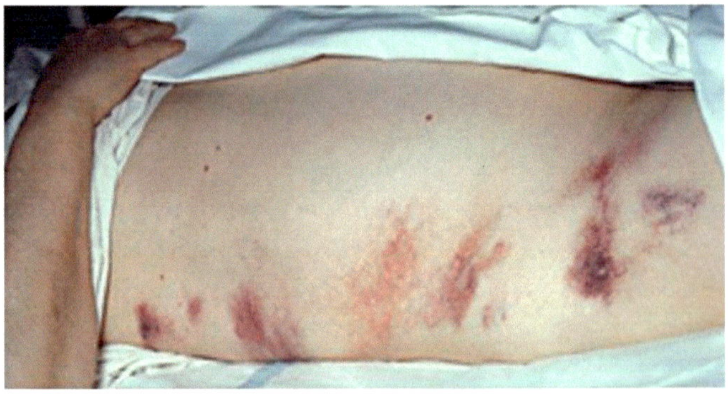

FIGURE 14.1.3 - Grey Turner Sign Suggesting Retroperitoneal Hemorrhage

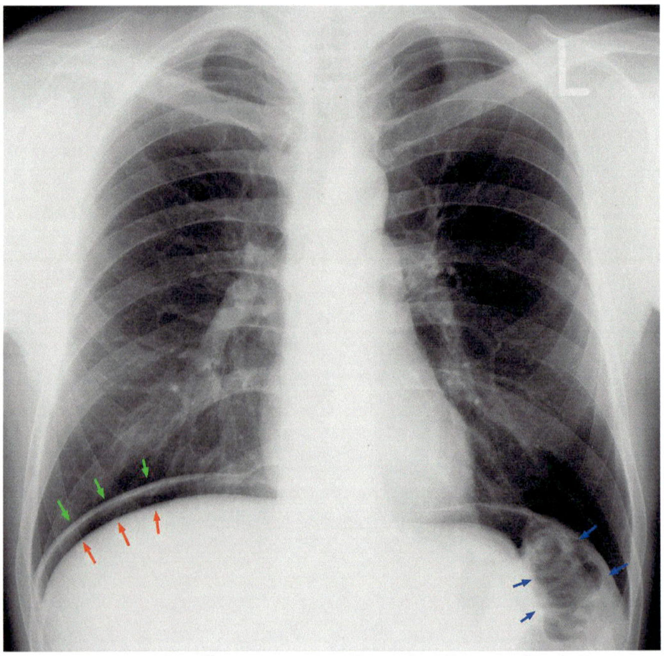

FIGURE 14.1.4 - Chest X-ray Showing Pneumoperitoneum

V. Blunt Abdominal Trauma: Diagnosis
   A. History and physical exam
   B. Imaging studies
      1. FAST ultrasound if hemodynamically unstable; investigates perihepatic and splenic spaces, pericardium, pelvis
      2. Radiography/CT scan if hemodynamically stable
      3. Diagnostic peritoneal lavage
      4. Laboratory workup: CBC, CMP, blood type and screen, and ABG

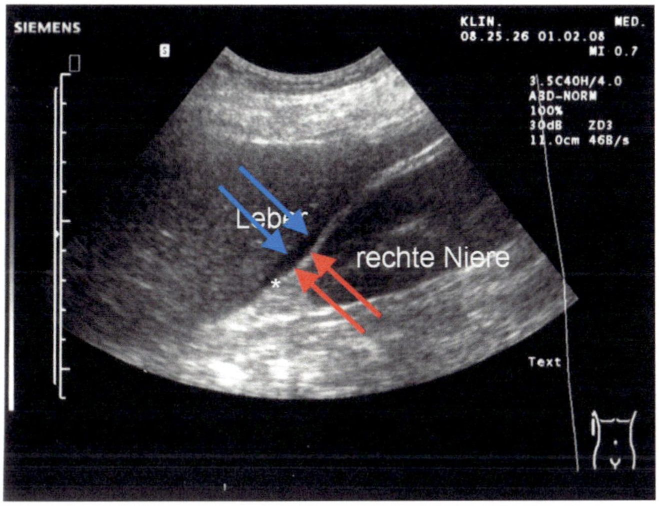

FIGURE 14.1.5 - FAST Image Showing Fluid in Morisson's Pouch (Space between Red and Blue Arrows)

VI. Blunt Abdominal Trauma: Management
   A. Primary survey (e.g. ABCDE system)
   B. Unstable patient → laparoscopy or laparotomy
   C. Stable patient with a normal primary survey → observation
   D. Stable patient with abdominal tenderness → abdominal/pelvic CT
   E. Secondary survey (e.g. history and physical exam)
   F. Diagnostic evaluation
   G. Most common cause of death in abdominal trauma → shock
   H. External bleeding → apply direct pressure
   I. Internal bleeding → IV fluids, blood transfusion, surgery
   J. Sepsis, peritonitis (hollow organ rupture) → antibiotic therapy, update tetanus status
   K. Assess patient first, then fetal status (e.g. airway, breathing, circulation, fetal HR)
   L. If unstable, give oxygen, IV access with fluid resuscitation, uterus displacement to the left if > 20 weeks
   M. CBC, type and screen, Kleihauer-Betke test if Rh-negative
   N. Fetal heart rate monitoring if viable, doppler auscultation if pre-viable
   O. Tocodynamometer

VII. Penetrating Abdominal Trauma: Definition/Etiology
   A. Gunshot wounds
      1. Small bowel, colon, liver, vessels
   B. Stab wounds
      1. Liver, small bowel, diaphragm, colon

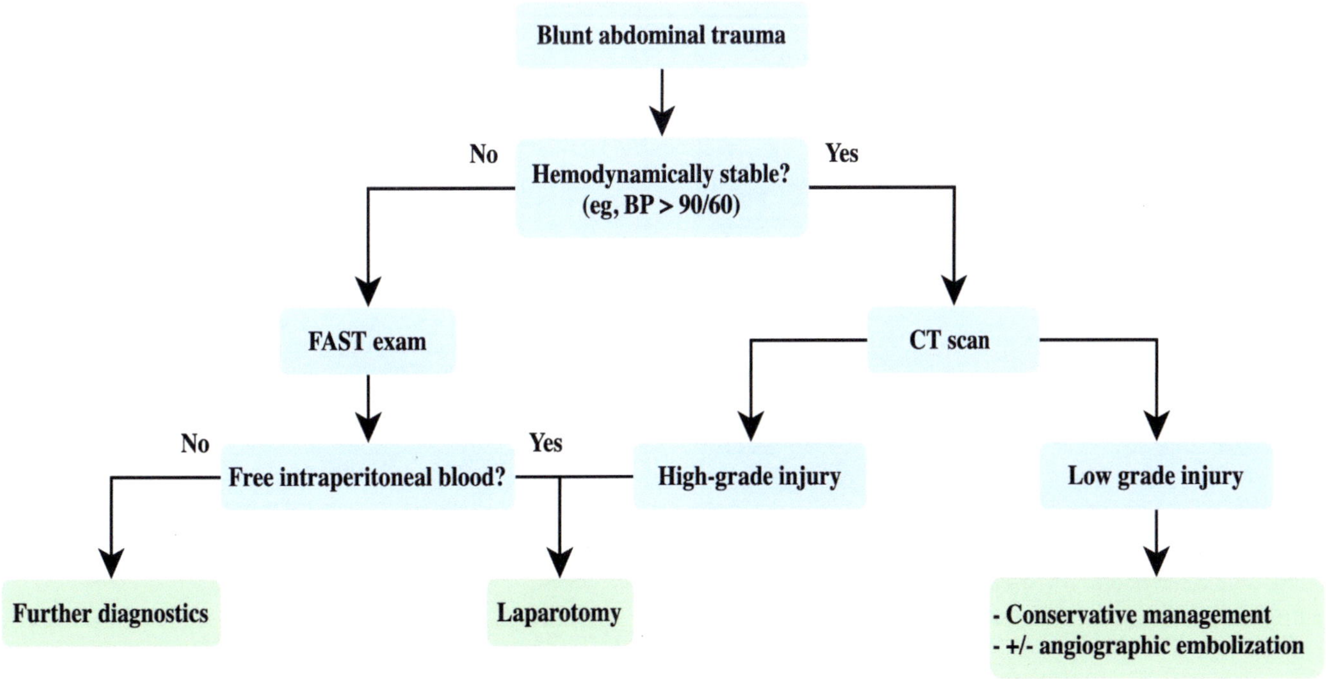

FIGURE 14.1.6 - Algorithm for Management of Blunt Abdominal Trauma

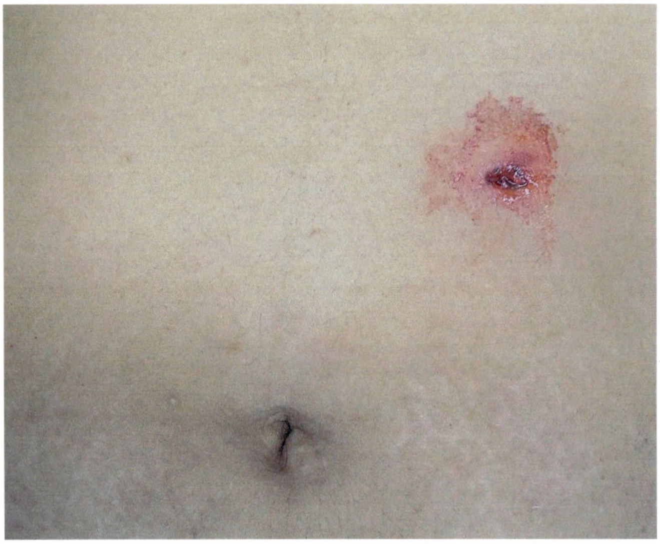

Bobjgalindo, CC BY-SA 4.0 <https://creativecommons.org/licenses/by-sa/4.0>, via Wikimedia Commons

FIGURE 14.1.7 - Gunshot Wound

VIII. Penetrating Abdominal Trauma: Clinical Features
- A. Abdominal pain
- B. Evisceration
- C. Bleeding or perforation
  - 1. May present with abdominal distension, altered levels of consciousness, peritoneal signs
- D. Shock
  - 1. Hypotension, tachycardia, changes in respiratory rate

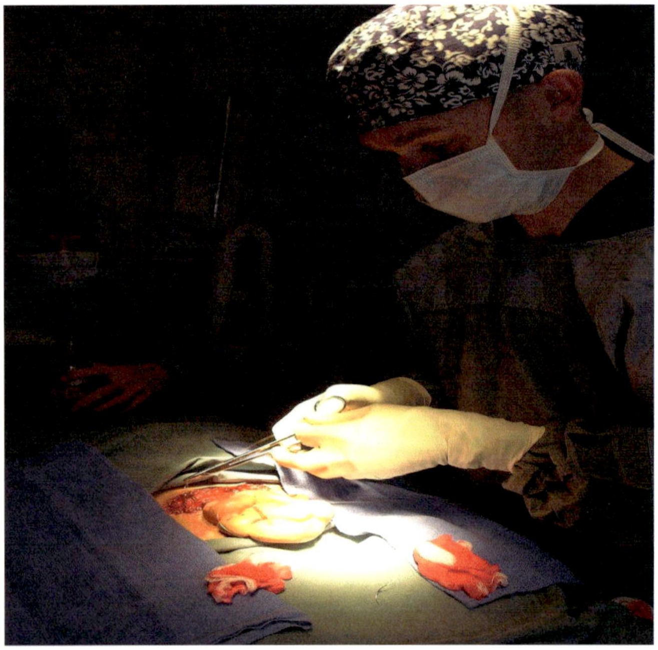

U.S. Navy photo by Lithographers Mate Seaman Rosa Shatusky, Public domain, via Wikimedia Commons

FIGURE 14.1.8 - Evisceration After Penetrating Abdominal Trauma

IX. Penetrating Abdominal Trauma: Diagnosis
- A. Clinical history and physical exam
- B. CBC, blood type, ABG
- C. BUN, creatinine, blood glucose, electrolytes, urinalysis
- D. Imaging, invasive procedures
  - 1. Stable: X-ray, CT
  - 2. Unstable: FAST, DPL (if FAST negative), diagnostic laparoscopy

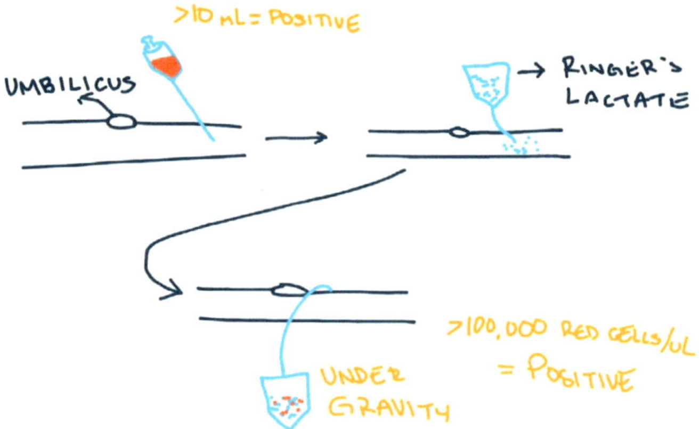

FIGURE 14.1.9 - Diagnostic Peritoneal Lavage

X. Penetrating Abdominal Trauma: Management
- A. ABCDE system
- B. IV fluids and blood transfusions as needed
- C. If unstable: laparotomy, antimicrobials, analgesics
- D. Urinary catheterization
- E. Nasogastric tube placement

Tests	Key Features
DPL	- Quick, early diagnosis - Invasive - Misses retroperitoneal and diaphragmatic injuries
FAST	- Quick, early diagnosis - Repeatable - Noninvasive - Can not assess for diaphragm and pancreatic injuries - Operator-dependent
CT scan	- Most specific - Sensitive - High cost and takes time - Needs transportation

TABLE 14.1.1 - Diagnostic Tests Used in Trauma Patients

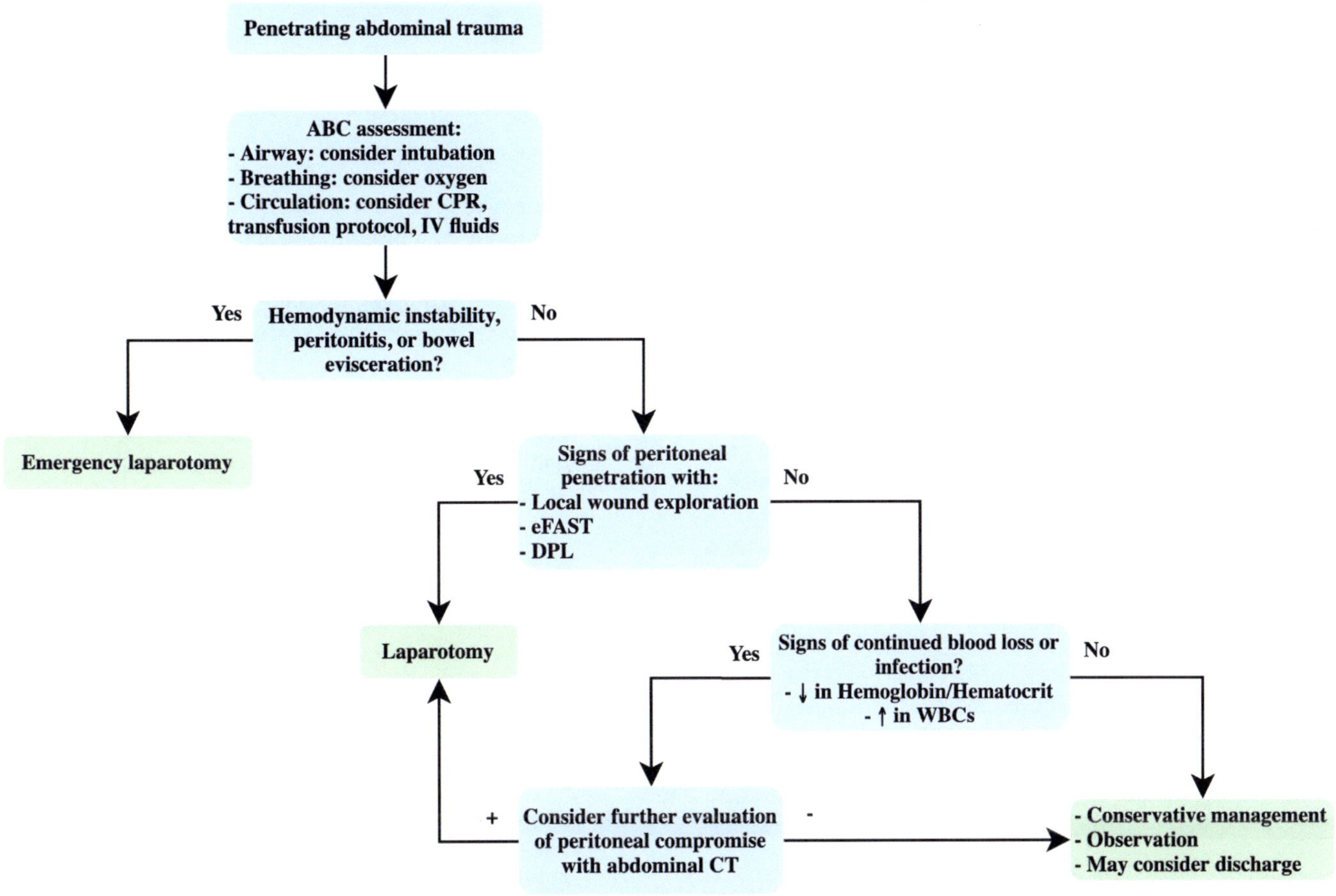

FIGURE 14.1.10 - Algorithm for Management of Penetrating Abdominal Trauma

REVIEW QUESTIONS

1. A 25-year-old gravid woman at 30 weeks gestation comes to the emergency department after a MVC, what is the best approach to this patient?

- **The best approach is an immediate consultation with obstetrics or transfer to a facility with those capabilities. Continuous fetal monitoring with a tocodynamometer should also be utilized. If the patient is stable and needs a CT scan then it can be done for pregnant trauma patients and is not associated with fetal anomalies. Nitrazine testing should be done to evaluate for rupture of membranes. A Kleihauer-betke test should be performed if the mother is O-negative in order to determine the amount of immunoglobulin that needs to be given to the mother if there has been exposure to the fetal blood.**
- It can be nerve-racking to have a pregnant trauma patient, but the basic principles of work up here are the same because what is good for the mother is what is good for the baby.
- As part of the circulatory evaluation, consideration must be given to the uterus compressing the vena cava which may be worsening the cardiac output.
- While maintaining C-spine precautions the uterus should be manually displaced to the left side.
- In making the decision of stable vs. unstable, keep in mind the vital sign changes associated with pregnancy.
- Pregnant patients have increased intravascular volume which allows them to lose a greater amount of blood volume before their heart rate or blood pressure will change- so the fetus may be in distress, due to the decreased perfusion to the placenta, despite the mother having normal vitals signs.
- During the abdominal exam evaluation for placental abruption or uterine rupture are critical, and these may or may not have vaginal bleeding associated with them.
- Immediate consultation with obstetrics is required or transfer to a facility with those capabilities.

2. In what scenarios would a diagnostic peritoneal lavage be indicated? In which scenario is DPL an absolute contraindication?

- **A diagnostic peritoneal lavage would be indicated for a penetrating abdominal trauma, if there is fascial penetration then a DPL is indicated. For blunt abdominal trauma if the patient is hemodynamically unstable and the FAST exam is not available, negative, or equivocal, then DPL is also indicated.**
- **Previous abdominal surgery is the only absolute contraindication due to the increased risk of damaging an organ or interference from adhesions. Relative contraindications include coagulopathies, advanced cirrhosis, and morbid obesity.**
- Historically, diagnostic peritoneal lavage was used to a greater extent than it is today because it has high accuracy for evaluating intraperitoneal hemorrhage and rupture of a hollow viscus.
- Now, it is less common due to the FAST exam and availability of CT scans.
- For penetrating trauma, if there is hemodynamic instability then the patient will go for a laparotomy.
- If the patient is hemodynamically stable and does not have peritoneal signs then the wound should be explored; if there is fascial penetration then a DPL is indicated.

REVIEW QUESTIONS

3. A 15-year-old man is brought via ambulance to the emergency department because of a gunshot wound to his abdomen that occurred 20 minutes ago. After initial resuscitative measures, the bullet was removed from the edge of the exit wound. What characteristics indicate the patient requires emergent laparotomy?

- **Key features that indicate the patient needs a laparotomy would include signs of evisceration, peritoneal signs, rectal bleeding, or bloody aspirate from a nasogastric tube.**
- If all of those are negative, but the patient continues to be hemodynamically unstable, then he will also qualify for exploratory laparotomy.

4. A 14-year-old man is brought via ambulance to the emergency department after doing belly flops into the local lake with friends 30 minutes ago. The patient became unresponsive after jumping down and landing on a rock directly under his abdomen. Vitals signs are notable for tachycardia and significant hypotension. On arrival he had a GCS of 8. After initial resuscitative measures, the patient remains hypotensive. A FAST exam is performed. Which findings on the FAST exam would indicate a need for emergent laparotomy?

   A. Anechoic stripe in Morrison's pouch
   B. Anechoic collection in the pericardial sac
   C. No echogenic changes
   D. Ovoid anechoic lesion with few septa and no wall thickening of the liver
   E. Echogenic foci in the gallbladder

- **The correct answer is option A.**
- This patient has had major abdominal trauma and continues to be unstable despite resuscitative measures.
- The finding on a FAST exam that would indicate the need for a laparotomy in an unstable patient is any evidence of free fluid.
- Fluid is going to appear black, or anechoic, on ultrasound.
- Morrison's pouch refers to the space between the liver and kidney where intra-abdominal fluid will collect, so an anechoic stripe in Morrison's pouch indicates there is free fluid in the abdomen and this patient needs to go for a laparotomy.
- Option B is incorrect because an anechoic collection in the pericardial sac is consistent with the pericardial effusion or cardiac tamponade.
- Cardiac tamponade necessitates pericardiocentesis, not a laparotomy.
- Option C is incorrect because it is describing a normal fast exam.
- Option D is incorrect because an ovoid anechoic lesion with few septa and no wall thickening describes a liver cyst, which generally does not require treatment.
- Option E is incorrect because echogenic foci in the gallbladder are the sonographic description of gallstones, which is not an indication for laparotomy.

Emergency Medicine | Section 2: Chest Trauma - Aortic Injury & Cardiac Contusion

I. Aortic Injury: General Characteristics
   A. Rapid deceleration from blunt trauma produces shearing forces
   B. Most common site of the injury: aortic isthmus

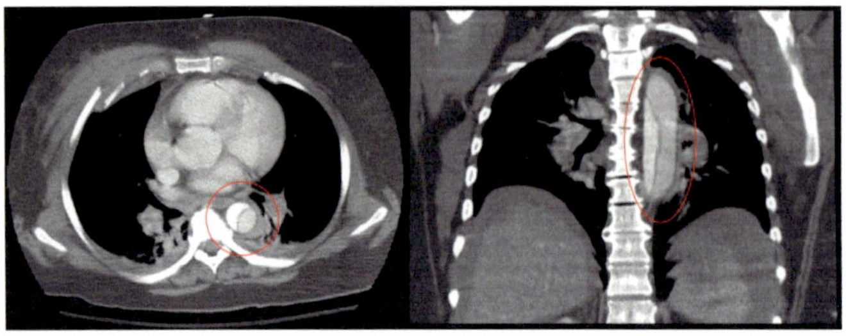

FIGURE 14.1.11 - CT of Chest with IV Contrast: Type B Aortic Dissection

II. Aortic Injury: Etiology
   A. Motor vehicle accidents
   B. Falls from heights

III. Aortic Injury: Clinical Features
   A. Chest pain, dyspnea
   B. Interscapular pain, dysphagia
   C. Physical exam findings
      1. Absent femoral pulses
      2. Interscapular murmur
      3. Hypertension (upper body)
      4. Left subclavian hematoma

IV. Aortic Injury: Diagnosis
   A. Chest CT (stable patients): intimal flap, hematoma, or aneurysm
   B. Chest X-ray: enlarged mediastinum, tracheal displacement, or hemothorax
   C. TEE (unstable patients): mediastinal hematomas, pseudoaneurysms, lacerations
   D. Aortography: location and type of the injury

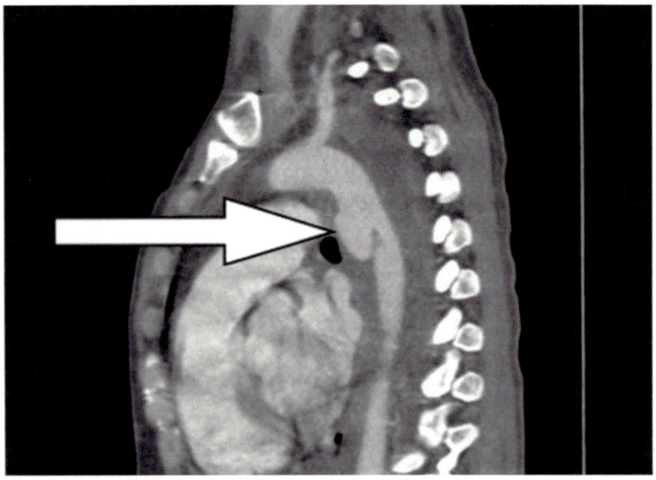

FIGURE 14.1.12 - CT of Chest: Saccular Aneurysm of Aorta

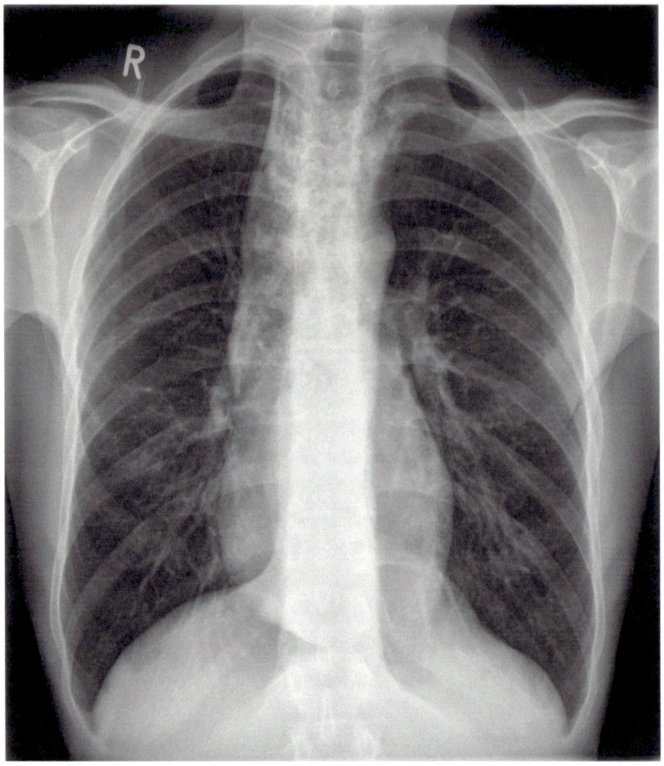

FIGURE 14.1.13 - Chest X-ray: Mediastinal Widening

V. Aortic Injury: Management
   A. Small intimal tear or small aortic hematoma
      1. Conservative management (e.g. blood pressure monitoring)
   B. Larger injuries or complete tears
      1. Open surgical repair
      2. Endovascular stent therapy

VI. Cardiac Contusion: General Characteristics
   A. Bruising of the myocardium due to decelerating force, direct or indirect pressure to the chest wall
   B. Can lead to LV dysfunction and cardiogenic shock
   C. Blow to the chest wall most commonly impacts the right ventricle

VII. Cardiac Contusion: Etiology
   A. Chest compressions
   B. Motor vehicle accidents
   C. Fall from height

VIII. Cardiac Contusion: Clinical Features
   A. Pain above ribs
   B. Bruising over the chest and upper abdomen
   C. Nausea, vomiting
   D. Dyspnea
   E. Arrhythmias
   F. Tachycardia

IX. Cardiac Contusion: Diagnosis
   A. 12-lead ECG: arrhythmias or ST changes

X. Troponins: Myocardial Injury
   A. TTE, TEE: ejection fraction, wall motion, and valvular function

XI. Chest X-ray or CT: Injuries of Chest Wall
   A. Cardiac Contusion: Management
   B. Oxygen
   C. Chest tube placement
   D. Pericardiocentesis if signs of tamponade
   E. Follow ACLS protocol for life-threatening rhythm abnormalities
   F. Cardiac telemetry
   G. Surgical repair

REVIEW QUESTIONS ?

1. A 27-year-old man is brought into the emergency department via ambulance after a motor vehicle accident 20-minutes ago. On arrival at the emergency department he complained of crushing chest pain. Rated 10/10 in severity, located substernally and radiated to the back. Vitals signs are unremarkable. What would be the best imaging modality to order if the patient?
   - **The best imaging modality to order is a CT chest. If this patient were brought in unconscious, the best imaging modality would be a transesophageal echocardiography.**
   - Stable patient → CT of chest; unstable patient → TEE.
   - One of the risk factors for aortic injury is rapid deceleration injury such as in a car accident.
   - Additionally, the common symptoms of aortic dissection include chest pain and interscapular pain.

2. A patient with a history of recent myocardial infarction requiring numerous chest compressions returns to the emergency department and is later diagnosed with a cardiac contusion. What is the effect on cardiac function?
   - **Cardiac contusion causes myocardial injury leading to cardiac dysfunction.**
   - This patient recently required numerous chest compressions which causes acute myocardial injury secondary to blunt force trauma.
   - Cardiac contusion → myocardial injury → ↓ LV function → ↓ CO

3. A 25-year-old man who works as a professional athlete is brought to the emergency department via ambulance because of severe chest pain after being involved in a motor vehicle accident 30 minutes ago. Rapid deceleration led him to hit his chest against the steering wheel. Past medical history and family history are non-contributory. Vital signs include a temperature of 36° C (96.8° F), blood pressure of 80/60 mmHg, heart rate of 125 beats/min, and respiratory rate of 21 breaths/min. Physical examination shows a large bruise across his chest. ECG shows non-specific ST-T wave changes. Initial Troponin I is 1 ng/mL with 2-hour repeat of 0.8 ng/mL (< 0.04 ng/mL). CXR is unremarkable. Which of the following is the most likely diagnosis in this patient?

   A. STEMI
   B. Stable angina
   C. Unstable angina
   D. Myocardial contusion

   - **The correct answer is option D.**
   - This young athlete presents with severe chest pain after being involved in a motor vehicle accident 30 minutes ago.
   - Rapid deceleration led him to hit his chest against the steering wheel.
   - Vital signs are significant for hypotension with a blood pressure of 80/60 mmHg, tachycardia with a heart rate of 125 beats/min, and tachypnea evidenced by respiratory rate of 21 breaths/min.
   - Physical exam shows a large precordial bruise.
   - ECG shows non-specific ST-T wave changes.
   - Troponin I is 1 ng/mL with a 2-hour repeat of 0.8 ng/mL.
   - All these findings within the context of chest trauma in a young patient suggest the diagnosis of myocardial contusion.
   - Myocardial injury due to contusion can induce ECG changes and increased troponin levels.
   - Option A is incorrect because ST-elevation myocardial infarction, also known as STEMI, is characterized by ST elevation on ECG. This patient, in contrast, has non-specific ST-T wave changes.
   - Option B is incorrect because there is no troponin rise with stable angina.
   - Option C is incorrect because unstable angina does not lead to increased troponin levels.

Emergency Medicine | Section 3: Chest Trauma - Pulmonary Contusion & Diaphragmatic Rupture

I. Pulmonary Contusion: General Characteristics
   A. Injury to the lung parenchyma, most commonly from blunt trauma, leading to lung consolidation and collapse secondary to edema and blood accumulation in the alveoli
   B. Hypoxic pulmonary vasoconstriction
      1. Attempt to prevent V/Q mismatch

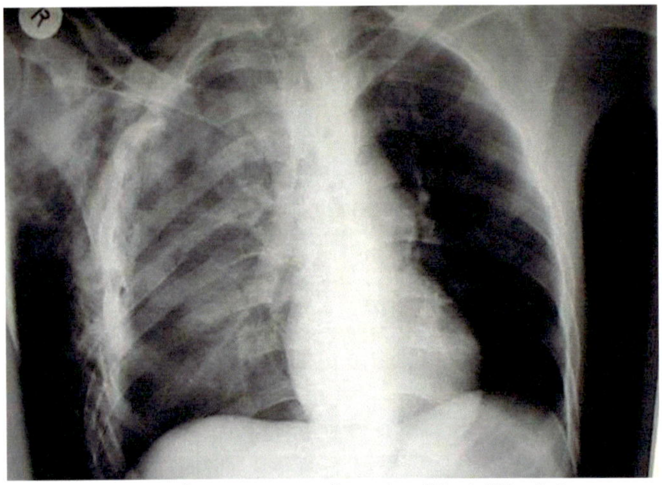

FIGURE 14.1.14 - Chest X-ray: Pulmonary Contusion

II. Pulmonary Contusion: Etiology
   a. Blunt trauma (e.g. rapid deceleration, sports injury, falls)
   b. Penetrating trauma
   c. Localized lesions (e.g. fractured ribs)
   d. Lung tissue shearing

III. Pulmonary Contusion: Clinical Features
   A. Dyspnea, hemoptysis, wheezing
   B. Hypotension, tachycardia, tachypnea
   C. Decreased breath sounds
   D. May be asymptomatic initially and can develop signs slowly

IV. Pulmonary Contusion: Diagnosis
   A. Chest X-ray
      1. Pulmonary changes may take 24 - 48 hours to be visible
      2. Will show irregular opacifications or diffuse opacifications (white out)
   B. CT scan
      1. May show better resolution of the injury

V. Pulmonary Contusion: Management
   A. Oxygen therapy
   B. CPAP, BiPAP
   C. Intubation, mechanical ventilation
   D. Pain control
   E. Chest physiotherapy
   F. Optimal positioning

VI. Diaphragmatic Rupture: General Characteristics
   A. Usually secondary to blunt or penetrating trauma
   B. Anterior compression
   C. Lateral compression
      1. Posterolateral diaphragm is weakest point
   D. Most diaphragmatic injuries occur on the left side as the right side is protected by liver

VII. Diaphragmatic Rupture: Etiology
   A. Penetrating injury (e.g. gunshots, stab wounds)
   B. Blunt trauma (e.g. motorcycle and car accidents)

VIII. Diaphragmatic Rupture: Clinical Features
   A. Dyspnea, chest pain, abdominal pain
   B. Nausea, vomiting
   C. Physical exam findings
      1. Displacement of abdominal organ into the thorax
      2. Bowel sounds on cardiac, lung auscultation
      3. Decreased breath sounds
      4. Scaphoid abdomen

IX. Diaphragmatic Rupture: Diagnosis
   A. FAST: large tears through the diaphragm, eviscerated organs
   B. Chest X-ray: elevated diaphragm, gastric or colonic bubble in the left chest, coiled NGT, rib fracture, pneumoperitoneum
   C. If the chest X-ray is non-diagnostic or abnormal → CT scan

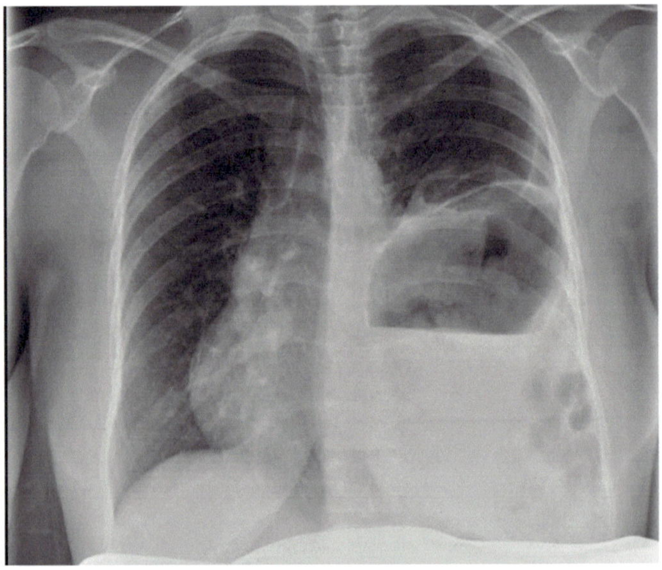

FIGURE 14.1.15 - Chest X-ray: Diaphragmatic Rupture

X. Diaphragmatic Rupture: Management
   A. IV fluids if hypotensive
   B. Pain control
   C. Exploratory laparoscopy, laparotomy

REVIEW QUESTIONS

1. How can a chest X-ray be used to differentiate between pulmonary contusion and a pneumothorax?
    - **In the setting of a pulmonary contusion, a chest X-ray would show diffuse opacification (white off) because edema and/or blood accumulate in the alveolar spaces. While a pneumothorax, would show loss of lung markings secondary to lung collapse.**
    - Contusion → consolidation; pneumothorax → loss of lung markings, collapsed visceral pleura.

2. A 35-year-old man is brought via ambulance to the emergency department because of a motorcycle accident 30 minutes ago. Physical examination is notable for bowel sounds when auscultating the heart. What additional findings would you expect in this patient on examination of the lungs?
    - **Additional findings on lung examination would likely be decreased breath sounds as the lungs have less room in the thorax as abdominal contents are now in the thorax.**
    - Based on the recent motorcycle accident paired with the finding of bowel sounds in the chest region, a ruptured diaphragm is suspected.
    - A ruptured diaphragm means there is no longer an acting barrier separating the abdominal viscera from the thorax, this allows contents to be displaced superiorly.
    - Abdominal viscera in thorax → ↓ breath sounds + scaphoid abdomen.

3. A 28-year-old man is brought to the emergency department because of severe chest and abdominal pain after being involved in a motorcycle accident 1 hour ago. His past medical history is non-contributory. Vital signs include temperature of 98.6° F (37° C), blood pressure of 100/70 mmHg, heart rate of 92 beats/min, and respiratory rate of 25 breaths/min. Physical examination shows a scaphoid abdomen along with bowel sounds on lung auscultation. ECG is unremarkable and cardiac troponin I is normal. Intravenous normal saline is initiated, and a FAST exam has been performed. Which of the following is the next best step in the diagnosis of this patient?

    A. Chest X-ray
    B. Chest CT scan
    C. PET scan
    D. PET-CT scan

    - **The correct answer is option A.**
    - This young man presents with severe chest and abdominal pain after being involved in a motorcycle accident 1 hour ago.
    - Vital signs are significant for tachypnea with the respiratory rate of 25 breaths/min.
    - Physical examination is notable a scaphoid abdomen along with bowel sounds on lung auscultation.
    - These findings are classic for a diaphragmatic rupture.
    - Intravenous normal saline is initiated to support the patient's hemodynamic status, and FAST exam has been performed.
    - The best next step in the diagnosis of the diaphragmatic rupture is a chest X-ray.
    - Chest X-ray typically shows an elevated diaphragm and a gastric or colonic bubble in the left hemithorax. It may also show pneumoperitoneum or rib fracture.
    - Option B is incorrect because chest CT scan is only performed in patients with suspected diaphragmatic rupture and the chest X-ray is non-diagnostic or abnormal.
    - Options C and D are incorrect because PET scan and PET-CT scan are not indicated in a patient with diaphragmatic rupture.

Emergency Medicine | Section 4: Chest Trauma - Flail Chest & Penetrating Chest Injury

I. Flail Chest: General Characteristics
   A. At least 2 fractures per rib in at least adjacent ribs
   B. Paradoxical chest movement
      1. Flail chest segment is sucked in with inspiration
      2. Flail chest segment is ballooned out outwards with expiration

II. Flail Chest: Etiology
   A. Motor vehicle collisions (most common)
   B. Falls (e.g. elderly)
   C. Chest compression

III. Flail Chest: Clinical Features
   A. Dyspnea
   B. Pleuritic chest pain
   C. Tachypnea
   D. Physical exam findings
      1. Paradoxical chest wall movement

IV. Flail Chest: Diagnosis
   A. Physical exam
   B. Chest X-ray
   C. CT
   D. Arterial blood gas

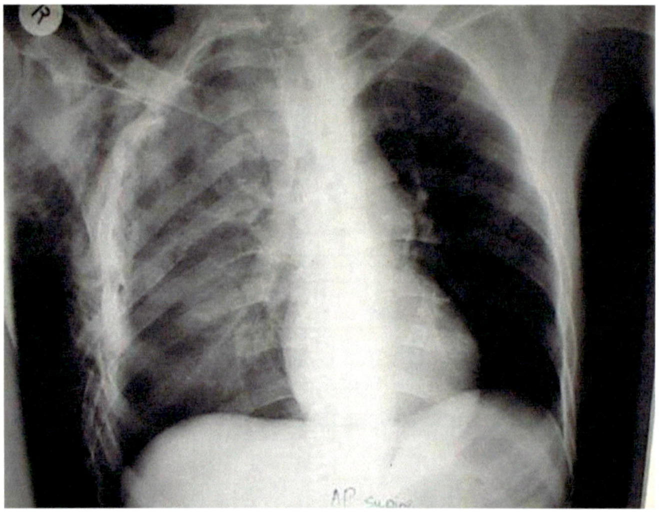

FIGURE 14.1.15 - Chest X-ray: Multiple Rib Fractures

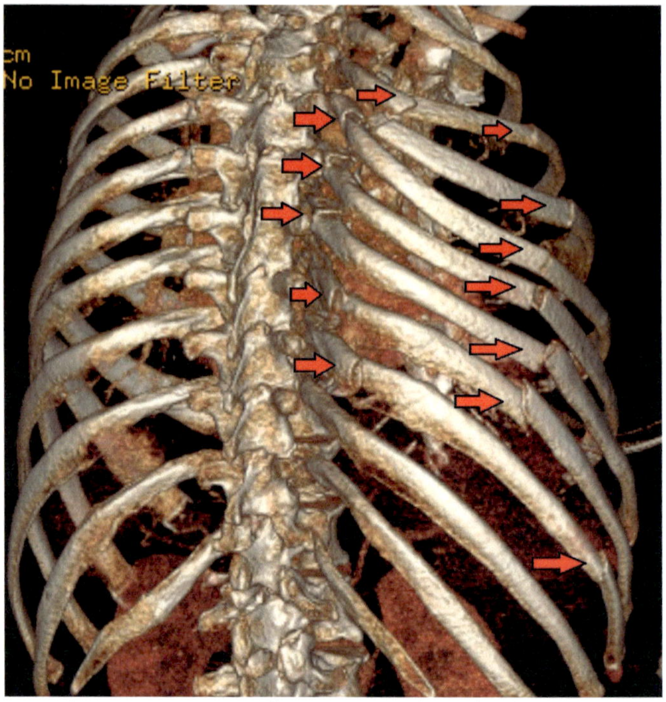

FIGURE 14.1.16 - Flail Chest

V. Flail Chest: Management
   A. Pain control
   B. Positive pressure ventilation
   C. Tube thoracostomy if pneumothorax occurs
   D. Surgical internal fixation
   E. Intubation
   F. Physiotherapy

VI. Penetrating Chest Injury: General Characteristics
   A. Open chest wound
   B. Hemothorax (blood accumulation in the pleural space)
   C. Pneumothorax (air entry into the chest)
   D. Cardiac tamponade (blood accumulation in the pericardial sac)
   E. Pneumomediastinum (air escapes from the lung or abdomen into mediastinum)

VII. Penetrating Chest Injury: Clinical Features
   A. Hemothorax: shock, tracheal deviation, dullness to percussion
   B. Pneumothorax: respiratory distress, decreased breath sounds, JVD, tracheal deviation, tachycardia, narrow pulse pressure, tympanic sounds on percussion
   C. Cardiac tamponade: Beck triad (JVD, hypotension, distant heart sounds), electrical alternans
   D. Pneumomediastinum: pleuritic chest pain, Hamman sign

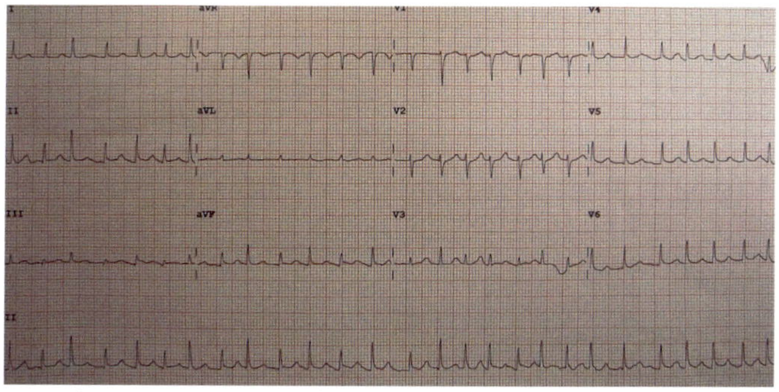

FIGURE 14.1.17 - ECG: Electrical Alternans

VIII. Penetrating Chest Injury: Diagnosis

A. ABC trauma evaluation for stability
B. ABG, CBC
C. FAST
D. Chest X-ray, CT
E. Echocardiogram

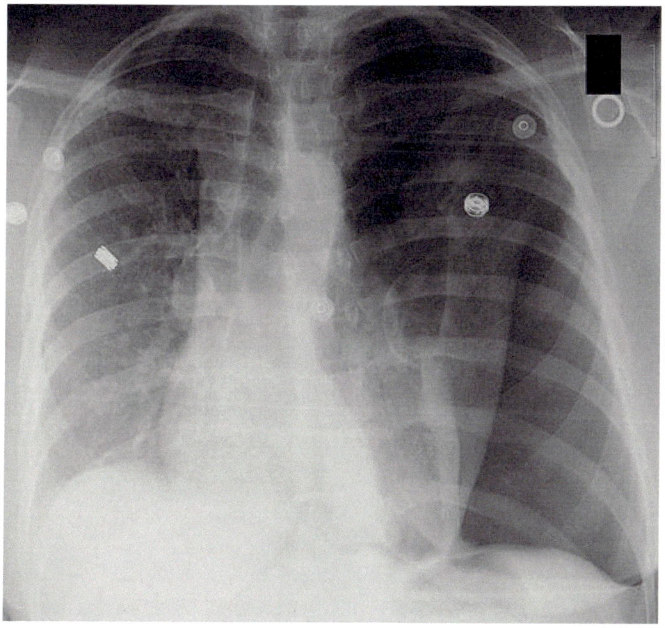

FIGURE 14.1.18 - Chest X-ray: Tension Pneumothorax

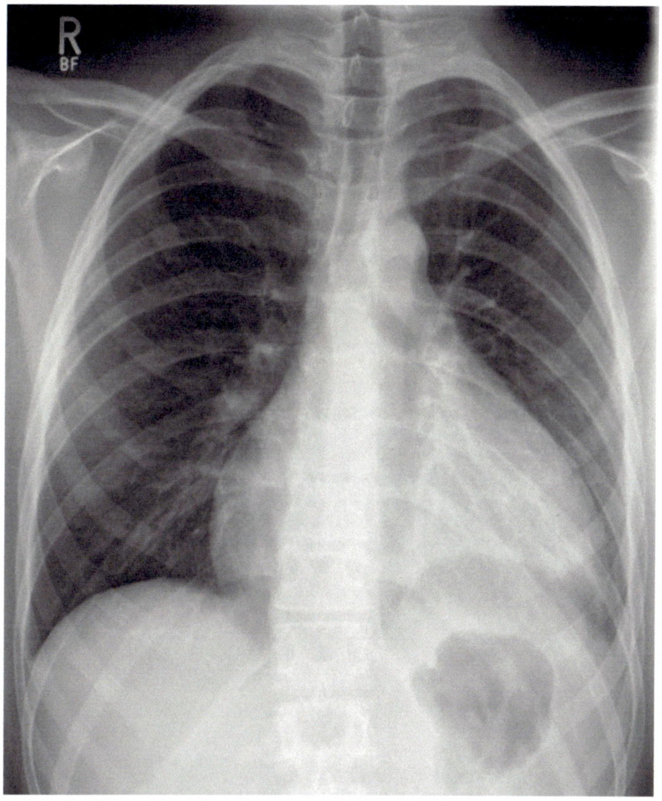

FIGURE 14.1.19 - Chest X-ray: Cardiomegaly

IX. Penetrating Chest Injury: Management

A. Needle thoracostomy, tube thoracostomy
B. Pericardiocentesis
C. IV fluids
D. Stable
   1. Echocardiogram
   2. Observation
E. Sternotomy, thoracotomy

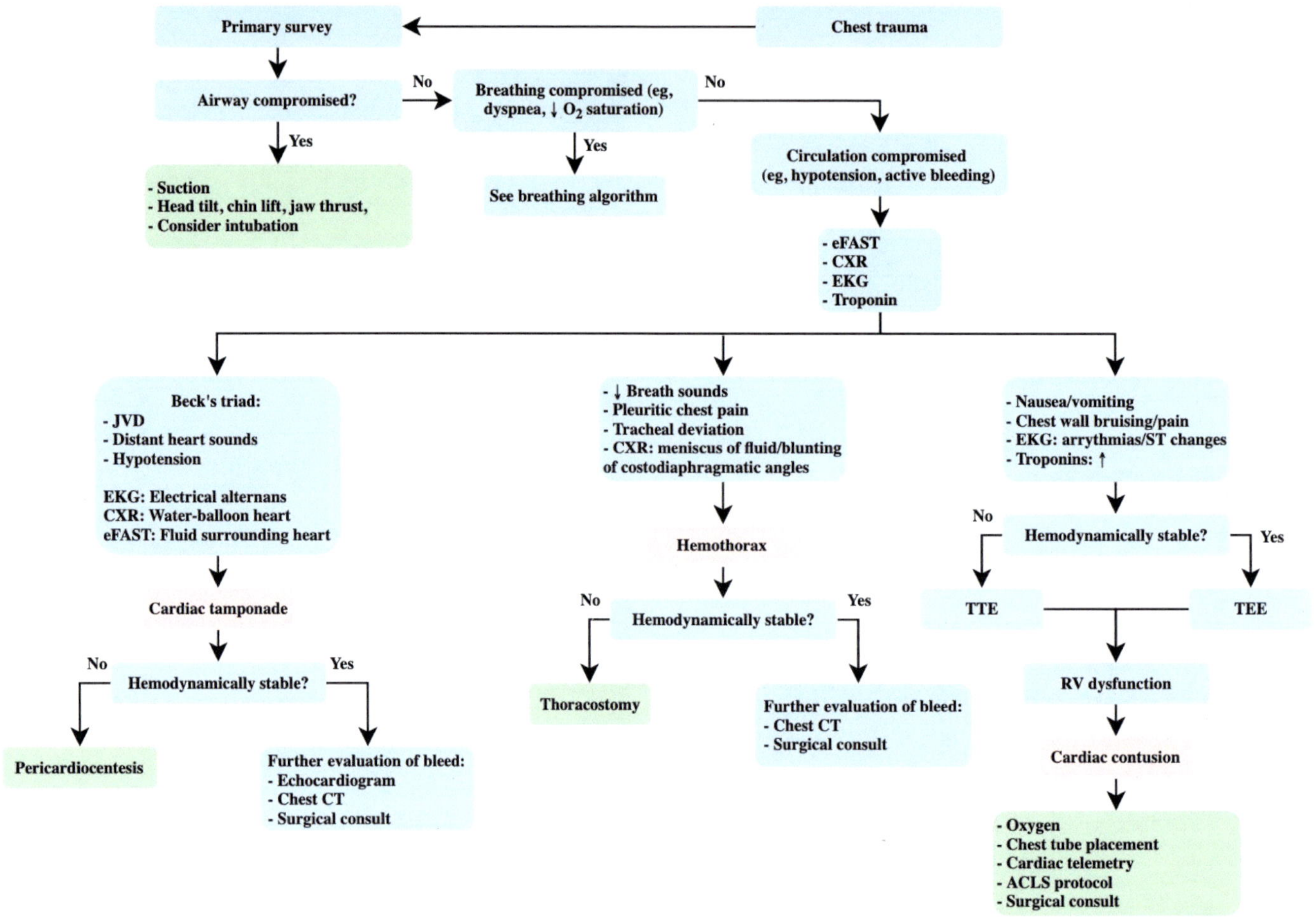

FIGURE 14.1.20 - Diagnosis and Management of Chest Trauma

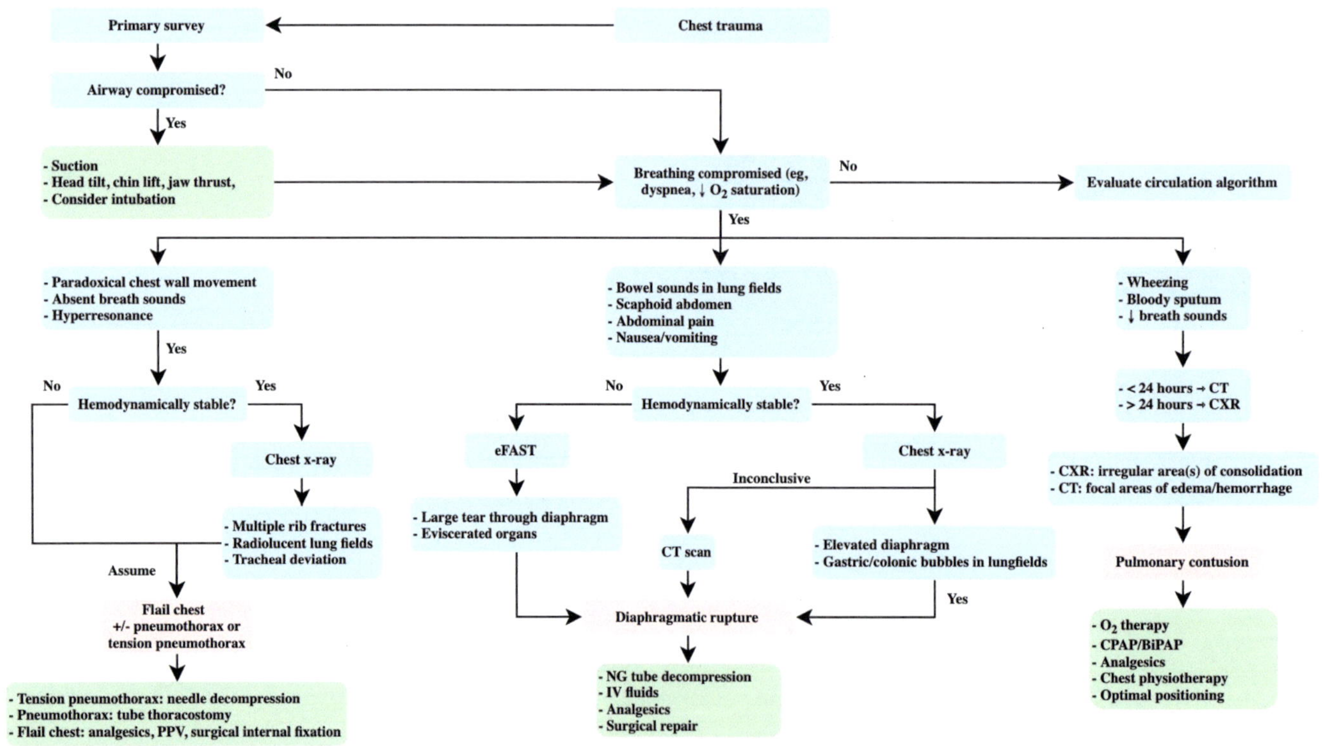

FIGURE 14.1.21 - Diagnosis and Management of Chest Trauma with Difficulty Breathing

REVIEW QUESTIONS

1. A 25-year-old man is brought to the emergency department via ambulance following a motor vehicle accident that occurred 30 minutes ago. On arrival he had chest pain and significant shortness of breath. Initial chest X-ray shows fractures in ribs 4 - 6 on the patient's right side with two fractures per rib. What is the characteristic physical exam finding likely to be seen in this patient?

   - **The characteristic physical exam finding likely to be seen in this patient is paradoxical chest movement (flail chest): when the patient inhales, the chest wall is pulled inwards; when the patient exhales, the chest wall is pushed outwards.**
   - This patient presents to the emergency department following a motor vehicle accident and is complaining of chest pain and dyspnea.
   - Chest X-ray shows fractures in ribs 4-6 on the patient's right side with two fractures per rib, which is consistent with flail chest.
   - The characteristic physical exam finding in flail chest is paradoxical chest movements meaning the chest wall will move opposite that of a healthy patient during respiration.
   - When the patient inhales, the chest is pulled inwards instead of outwards. Additionally, when the patient exhales, the chest wall will be pushed outwards instead of inwards.

2. During a play rehearsal an actor is accidentally 'stabbed' in the right upper chest with what was assumed to be a fake spear. On chest X-ray, there is an absence of peripheral lung markings on the right side and the trachea is shifted to the left. Based on the type of injury and chest X-ray findings, what would be expected on auscultation and percussion of this patient?

   - **Based on the type of injury and chest X-ray findings, decreased breath sounds on auscultation and tympanic sounds on percussion would be expected.**
   - This patient has a penetrating chest injury which has allowed air inside of the pleural cavity, thus making the intrapleural pressure equal to the atmospheric pressure and collapsing the right lung. This is the definition of a pneumothorax.
   - The chest X-ray findings of absent peripheral lung markings help to distinguish this injury from a hemothorax, which is typically associated with opacification of the thorax on the affected side secondary to blood accumulation.
   - On auscultation of a pneumothorax, since the right lung is collapsed, decreased or absent breath sounds on the right side is expected. On percussion, since the right lung is deflated and there is a significant amount of air in the chest, louder tympanic sound is expected.
   - This is in contrast to a hemothorax, where one would expect to hear decreased breath sounds and dull sounds on percussion.

REVIEW QUESTIONS

3. A 48-year-old man is brought to the emergency department via ambulance because of a stab wound to the left side of his chest. He was attacked roughly 30-minutes ago. The patient is A&Ox3, but is moaning in pain. Vital signs include temperature of 98.6° F (37° C), blood pressure of 80/50 mmHg, heart rate of 150 beats per minute, and respiratory rate of 25 breaths per minute. SaO_2 on room air is 97%. Physical examination shows jugular venous distension and distant heart sounds. ECG shows low-voltage QRS complexes with alternating amplitudes. What is the next best step in the management of this patient?

    A. Pericardiocentesis
    B. IV normal saline
    C. Chest tube placement
    D. Intubation

- **The correct answer is option A.**
- This patient presents with a stab wound to the left side of the anterior chest wall.
- He is A&Ox3, but is moaning in pain.
- The patient is hemodynamically unstable, evidenced by the blood pressure of 80/50 mmHg, heart rate of 150 beats per minute, and respiratory rate of 25 breaths per minute.
- Physical examination shows jugular venous distension and distant heart sounds.
- Therefore, this patient has Beck's triad, which includes hypotension, jugular venous distension, and muffled heart sounds. Beck's triad is characteristic of cardiac tamponade.
- ECG shows low-voltage QRS complexes with alternating amplitudes. This sign is known as electrical alternans and is pathognomonic for the cardiac tamponade.
- The best next step in the management of an unstable patient with cardiac tamponade is emergent pericardiocentesis. It relieves the external pressure on the heart chambers and restores the end-organ perfusion.
- Option B is incorrect because although intravenous normal saline is promptly administered in the emergency department to maintain the end-organ perfusion, this patient is unstable and requires immediate stabilization with pericardiocentesis. Additionally, the patient's low blood pressure is a result of fluid in the pericardial sac compressing the heart, decreasing cardiac output. Normal saline will not impact the cardiac output, and will therefore not impact the blood pressure in this patient. The only option to improve their cardiac output is to remove the fluid to improve pumping function of the heart.
- Option C is incorrect because chest tube placement is used to treat pneumothorax, hydrothorax, hemothorax, and chylothorax. It is not useful in the management of cardiac tamponade.
- Option D, intubation, is incorrect because this patient has a secured airway evidenced by the normal oxygen saturation value of 97%.

Emergency Medicine | Section 5: Acute Appendicitis

I. Acute Appendicitis: Definition
   A. Obstruction of the appendiceal lumen leading to inflammation of the appendix
   B. Surgical emergency
   C. Early teens to middle-aged adults

II. Acute Appendicitis: Etiology
   A. Obstruction due to:
      1. Hyperplasia of lymphoid tissue (children)
      2. Fecalith (adults)
      3. Foreign body
      4. Parasites

III. Acute Appendicitis: Pathophysiology
   A. Obstruction leads to:
      1. Accumulation of bacteria due to stasis
      2. Distended appendix and intraluminal pressure exceeds the venous pressure causing vascular congestion
      3. Vascular supply compromised
      4. With ischemia, wall weakens and perforation occurs

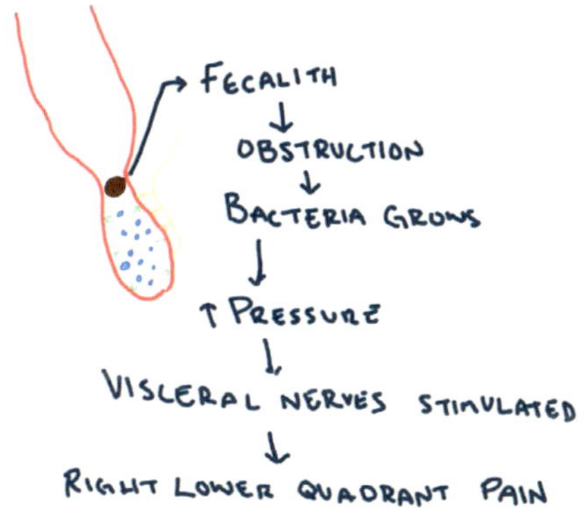

FIGURE 14.1.22 - Pathophysiology of Acute Appendicitis

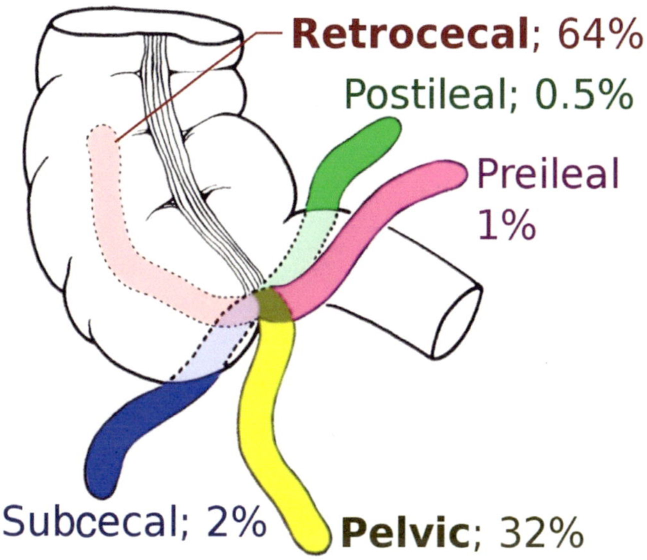

FIGURE 14.1.23 - Locations of Appendix

IV. Acute Appendicitis: Clinical Presentation
   A. Non-specific symptoms: anorexia, nausea, vomiting and fever
   B. Diarrhea or constipation
   C. Diffuse and dull periumbilical pain
   D. Localized sharp right lower quadrant pain (McBurney's point)
   E. Physical examination
      1. Pain at McBurney's point
      2. Rovsing sign
      3. Psoas sign
      4. Obturator sign
   F. Pseudoappendicitis
      1. Presents like appendicitis but with bloody diarrhea
      2. Classically due to *Yersinia enterocolitica*
      3. Typically self-limited, but can be fatal in immunocompromised patients
      4. Treat with doxycycline if immunocompromised

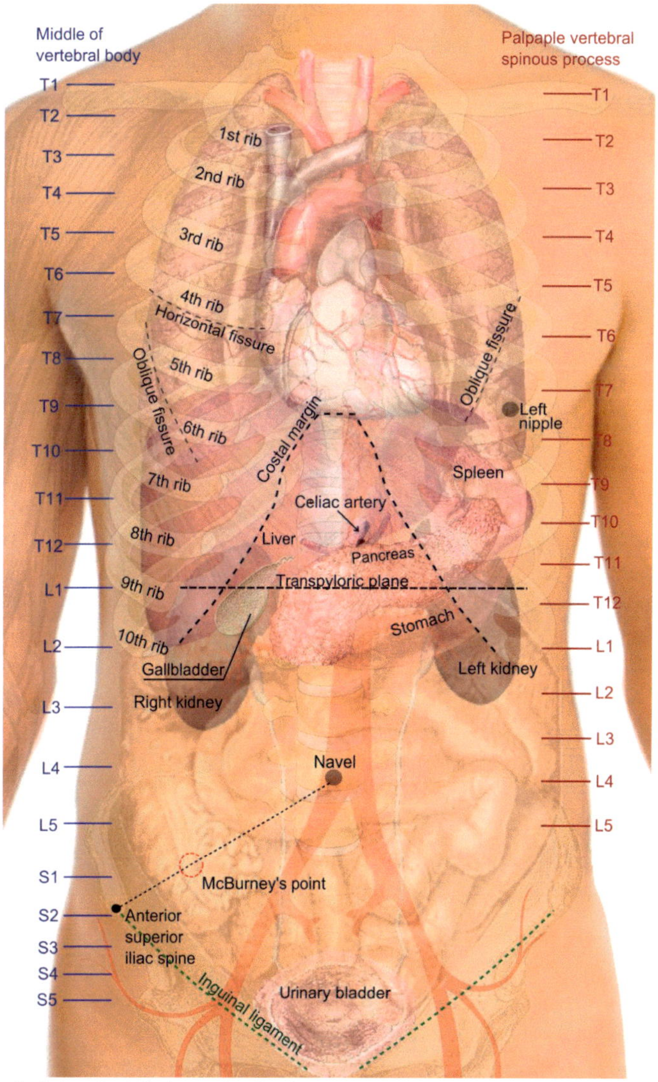

FIGURE 14.1.24 - McBurney's Point

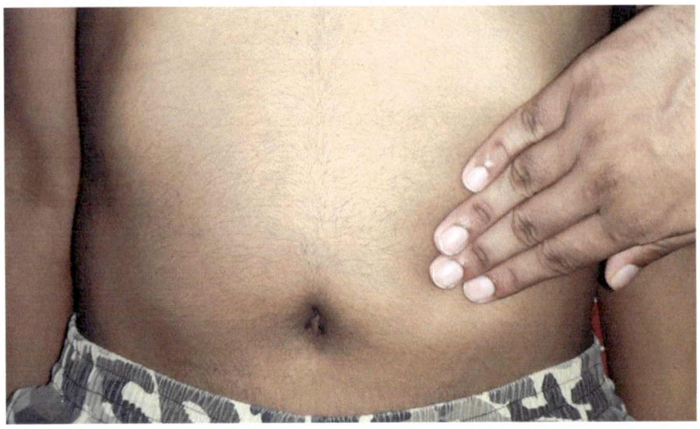

FIGURE 14.1.25 - Palpation of Left Lower Quadrant of Abdomen to Screen for Rovsing Sign

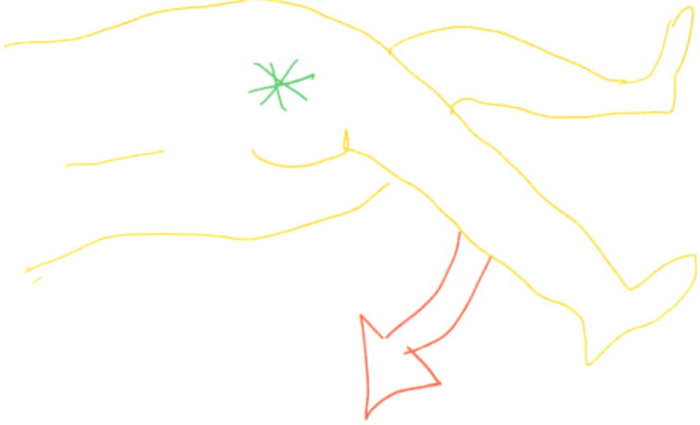

FIGURE 14.1.26 - Psoas Sign

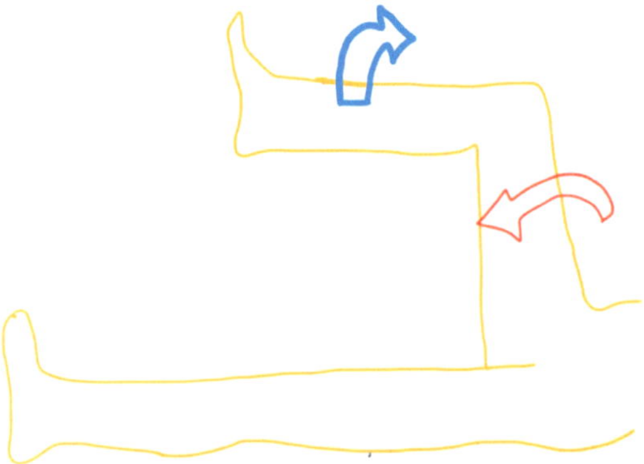

FIGURE 14.1.27 - Obturator Sign

V. Acute Appendicitis: Diagnosis
   A. Clinical: Alvarado scoring system
   B. Women of reproductive age with abdominal pain receive a beta-hCG pregnancy test to rule out ectopic pregnancy
   C. Leukocytosis with left shift, band cells
   D. Increased C-reactive protein
   E. Urinalysis: mild pyuria
   F. Imaging studies if uncertain
      1. CT scan with PO and IV contrast
         a) Enlarged appendix > 6 mm, fecalith, periappendiceal fat stranding, free fluid
      2. Ultrasound for children and pregnant women
         a) Enlarged appendix may be seen
         b) Peritoneal fluid or abscess in advanced cases

Alvarado score	
Feature	**Score**
Migration of pain	1
Anorexia	1
Nausea	1
Tenderness in right lower quadrant	2
Rebound pain	1
Elevated temperature	1
Leucocytosis	2
Shift of white blood cell count to the left	1
Total	**10**

TABLE 14.1.2 - Alvarado Score

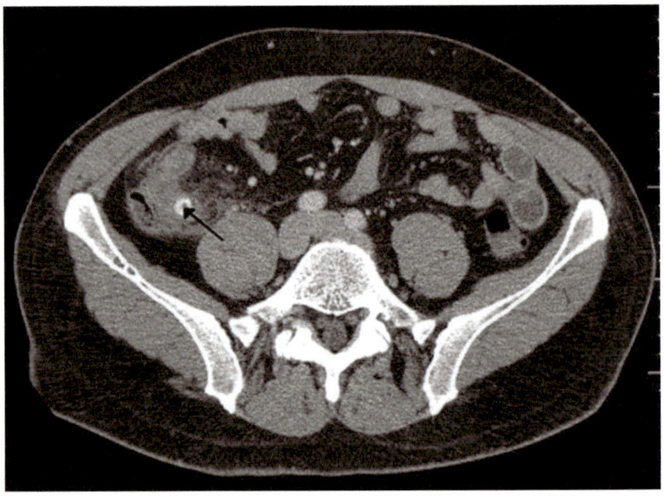

FIGURE 14.1.28 - CT Scan of Abdomen: Perforated Appendix

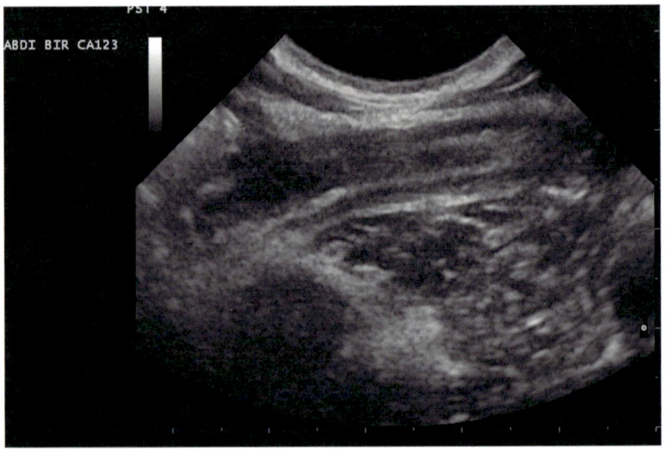

FIGURE 14.1.29 - Ultrasound of Abdomen: Acute Appendicitis

VI. Acute Appendicitis: Management
   A. Urgent open or laparoscopic appendectomy is definitive treatment
   B. NPO, IV fluids, analgesics, antiemetics
   C. Single dose of antibiotics covering anaerobic and gram negative bacteria
   D. Non-perforated appendicitis should not exceed antibiotic use over 24 hours

VII. Acute Appendicitis: Complications
   A. Perforated appendix
   B. Abscess formation
   C. Gangrenous appendicitis
   D. Inflammatory appendiceal mass
   E. Pylephlebitis

VIII. Perforated Appendix
   A. Free rupture of the appendix
   B. High fever, tachycardia, hypotension
   C. Rebound tenderness and guarding and decreased bowel sounds on physical examination
   D. Emergency appendectomy, intravenous antibiotics, give appropriate antibiotic once cultures are obtained

IX. Appendiceal Abscess
   A. Inflamed appendix surrounded by pus and necrotic tissue
   B. High grade fever, leukocytosis
   C. Localized RLQ pain and tenderness on physical examination
   D. Imaging: fluid collection surrounding appendix
   E. Abscess > 4 cm: drained → elective appendectomy 6 to 8 weeks later
   F. Abscess < 4 cm: antibiotics alone

X. Gangrenous Appendicitis
   A. Necrosis of the appendiceal wall
   B. Diagnosed intraoperatively
   C. High grade fever, tachycardia, tenderness
   D. Emergency appendectomy and intravenous antibiotics

XI. Inflammatory Appendiceal Mass
   A. Ill-defined mass of inflammatory periappendiceal tissue
   B. Tender mass localized in the right lower quadrant
   C. Intravenous antibiotics
   D. Surgery if no improvement after 48 hours of antibiotics

XII. Pylephlebitis
   A. Septic thrombosis of the portal vein or its branches that can lead to bowel infarction and death
   B. Sequelae of perforated appendicitis
   C. Fever, abdominal pain
   D. Broad spectrum antibiotics

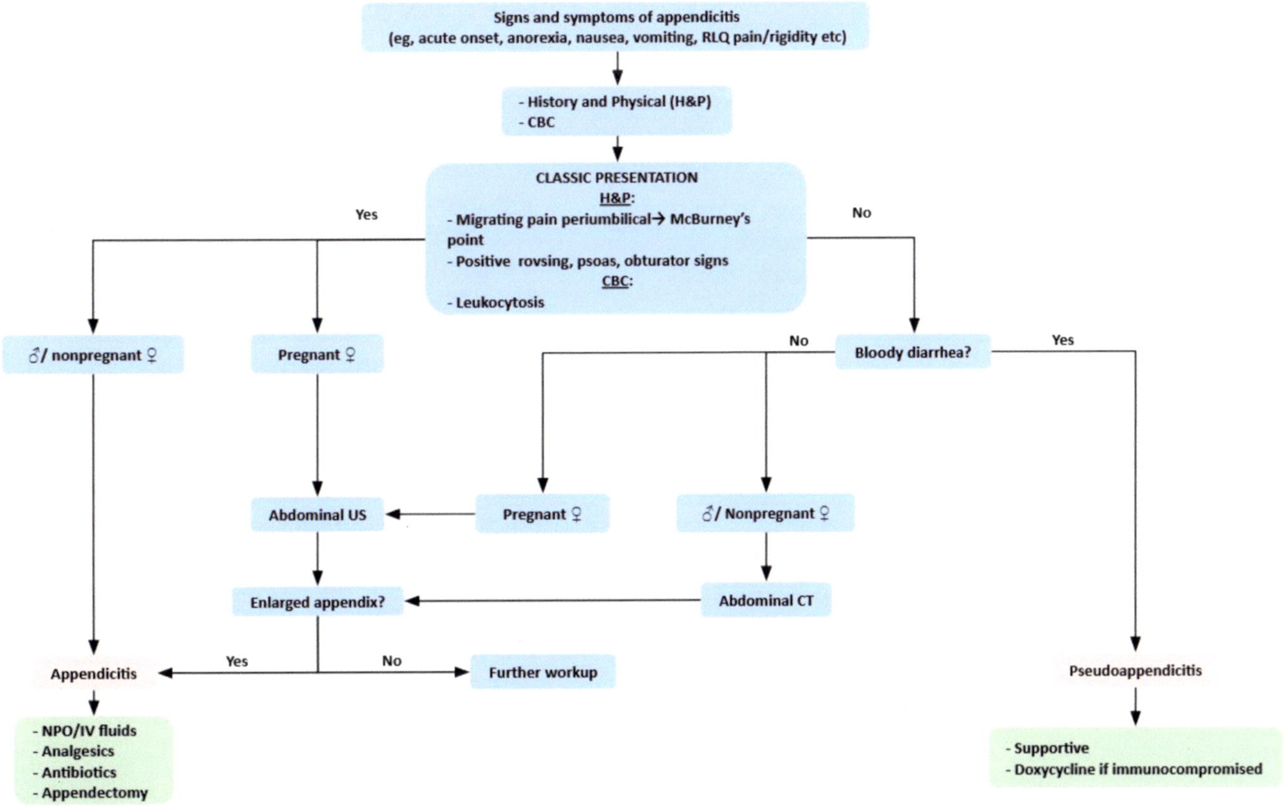

FIGURE 14.1.30 - Algorithm: Evaluation and Management of Acute Appendicitis

REVIEW QUESTIONS

1. How can a parasitic infection result in an abdominal abscess in the retrocecal area?

    - **A parasitic infection can result in an abdominal abscess in the following way: large parasite → obstruction → compromised vasculature → ischemia → perforation → abscess.**
    - A parasite(s) can become so large that they themselves cause obstruction, leading to vascular compromise.
    - The pathophysiology is similar to the process of a fecalith causing an obstruction.
    - The obstruction leads to distention and increased intraluminal pressure, thereby resulting in decreased venous system pressure, leading to vascular congestion and a compromised vascular supply leading to ischemia.
    - If left untreated, there is a weakening of the tissue wall which can result in perforation and potentially leading to abscess formation.

2. A 17-year-old obese woman is brought to the emergency department by her mother because of lower abdominal pain for the past 2-days. On physical examination there is significant right lower quadrant tenderness on palpation. She states the abdominal pain initially started at her belly button and has since moved to its current location. What diagnoses must you consider with this presentation and is any imaging warranted in this patient?

    - **Diagnoses considered with this presentation include appendicitis and ectopic pregnancy. In this patient, an ultrasound is warranted.**
    - This patient is presenting with concerns of appendicitis, especially due to the location of the pain and the age of the patient. However, before starting treatment of appendicitis, other life threatening conditions must be ruled out.
    - Ectopic pregnancy cannot be ruled out just by the history, so a urine pregnancy test must be done prior to imaging.
    - If a question describes a female patient with lower quadrant pain, a pregnancy test is always performed before ultrasound or CT scan to rule out ectopic pregnancy.
    - Then, if imaging is required, ultrasound is preferred for pregnant patients and children due to the contrast toxicity and radiation exposure that CT scans have.
    - Here ultrasound would be the preferred imaging.

3. A 27-year-old man comes to the emergency department because of abdominal pain for six days. Over the past 3 days he has also experienced nausea, and vomiting. Past medical history and family history is unremarkable. Vital signs show blood pressure of 90/60 mmHg, and pulse of 90 beats/min. Physical examination shows localized tenderness to palpation in the right lower quadrant. A CT scan of the abdomen is performed and shows a 3cm retrocecal well-defined fluid collection. Which of the following is the next best step in management after an IV fluid resusitation?

    A. Urgent laparotomy
    B. Proton pump inhibitors
    C. Intravenous antibiotics
    D. Analgesics

    - **The correct answer is option C.**
    - This patient presents with abdominal pain for almost a week.
    - Vitals signs reveal the patient is hypotensive and tachycardic.
    - Physical examination shows RLQ tenderness, which hints at appendicitis as a potential diagnosis.
    - CT scan is suspicious for abscess formation due to the defined retrocecal fluid collection.
    - In cases of appendiceal abscesses, IV antibiotics are indicated over surgery, making C the correct answer.
    - However, he should be stabilized from the standpoint of his hypotension first, which is why antibiotics would be given after an IV fluid bolus.
    - An appendiceal abscess must first be managed with intravenous antibiotics if it is less than 4 cm in size and drained percutaneously if the abscess is larger than 4 cm.
    - Morbidity and mortality is lower with this approach than with immediate surgery.
    - Option A is incorrect because urgent laparotomy is needed to prevent perforation, but since perforation has already occurred and resulted in abscess formation, IV antibiotics are indicated.
    - Option B is incorrect because proton pump inhibitors are a mainstay treatment for acute gastritis and peptic ulcer disease.
    - Option D is incorrect because although analgesics are given for pain management, the underlying condition needs to be addressed. Analgesics will be given, but intravenous antibiotics ultimately lowers the morbidity rate in patients with abscess formation from appendiceal rupture and will be the next best step in this case.

Emergency Medicine | Section 6: Abdominal Pain and Acute Abdomen

I. Abdominal Pain: Pathophysiology
   A. Visceral nerves: colicky pain, dull, and diffuse pain
   B. Somatic sensory nerves: sharp, localized pain with guarding
   C. Mechanical distension → rupture → leak in peritoneum → acute abdomen

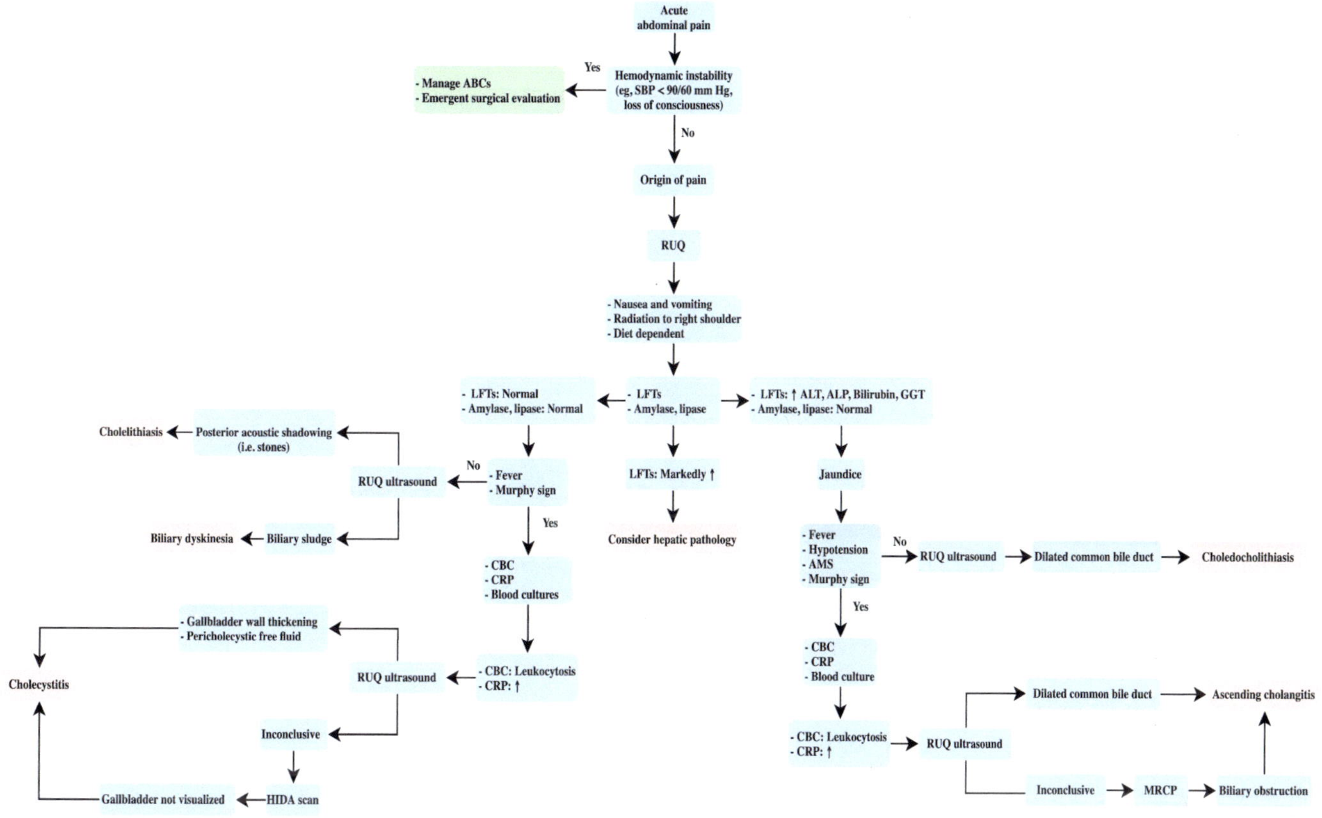

FIGURE 14.1.31 - Algorithm: Right Upper Quadrant Abdominal Pain

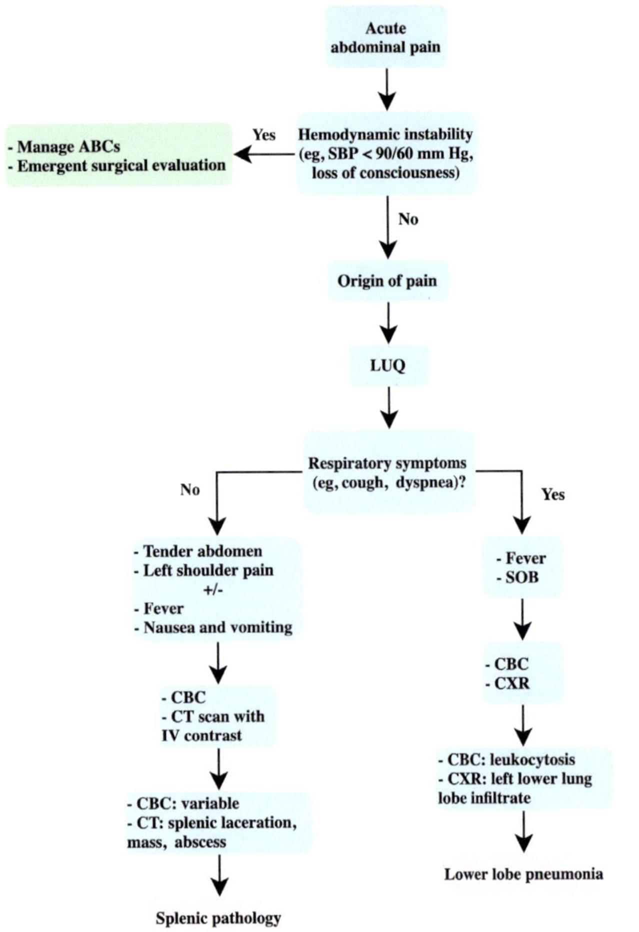

FIGURE 14.1.32 - Algorithm: Left Upper Quadrant Abdominal Pain

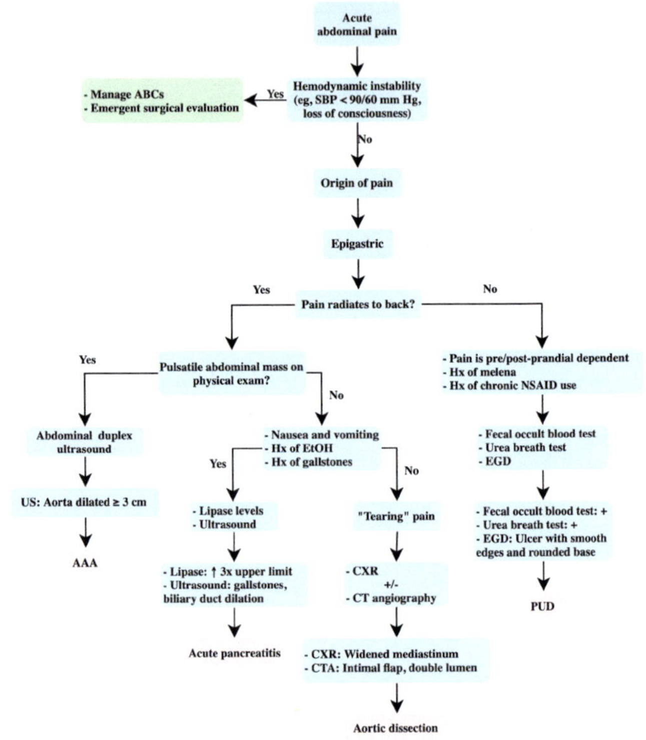

FIGURE 14.1.34 - Algorithm: Epigastric Abdominal Pain

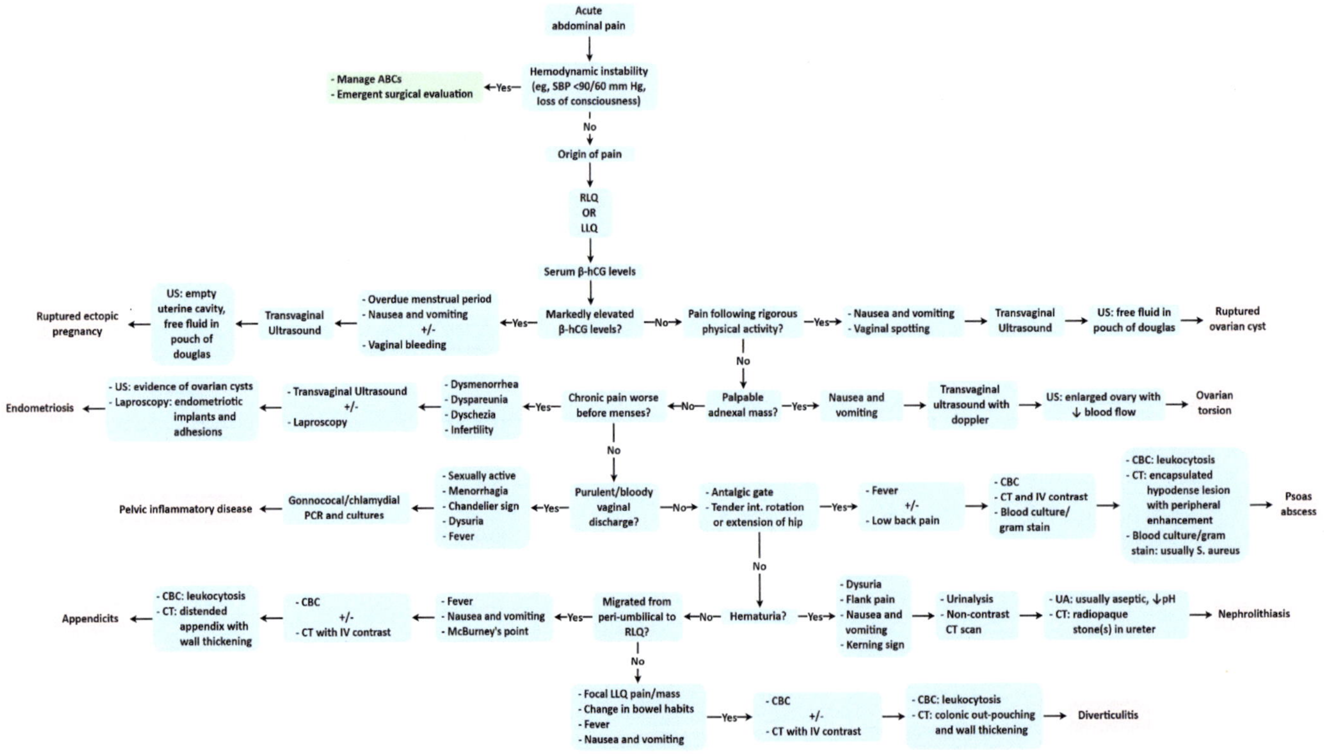

FIGURE 14.1.33 - Algorithm: Right Lower Quadrant and Left Lower Quadrant Abdominal Pain

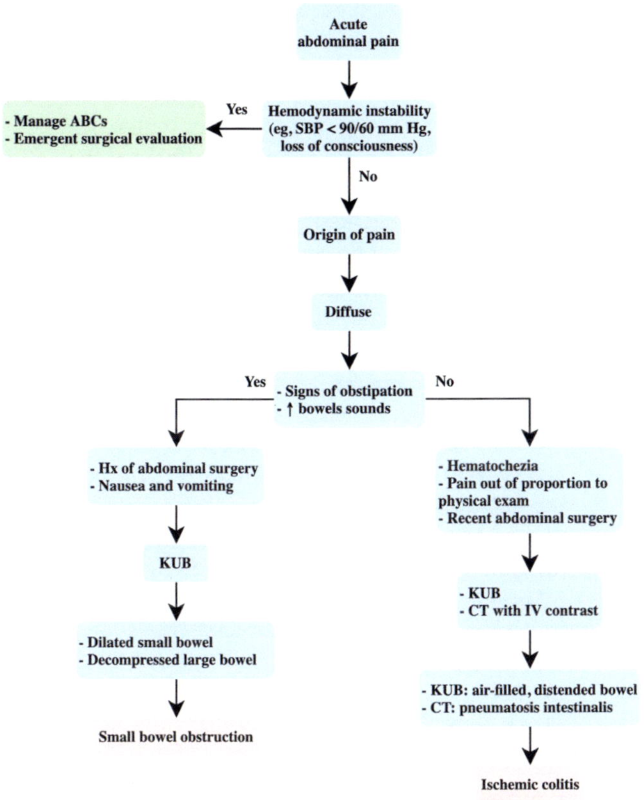

FIGURE 14.1.35 - Algorithm: Diffuse Abdominal Pain

II. Acute Abdomen
   A. Severe abdominal pain
   B. Acute onset < 5 days
   C. Thorough history and physical exam
   D. Peritoneal signs and shock call for immediate intervention
   E. Clinical diagnosis
   F. Tender abdomen with guarding and rigidity
   G. Absent bowel sounds
   H. Abdominal X-ray: free air under diaphragm
   I. If inconclusive, abdominal CT scan confirms diagnosis
   J. Pelvic ultrasound if positive β-hCG
   K. Hemodynamically unstable patient
      1. Emergent laparotomy
   L. Stable patient
      1. Treat underlying cause
      2. NPO, NGT, IV fluids, Foley catheter, abdominal exams, serial scans
      3. Parenteral analgesics and antiemetics, empiric antibiotic therapy

REVIEW QUESTIONS

1. A 45-year-old G5P5 woman was brought to the emergency department by her partner because of abdominal pain for the past 4 hours. She has had similar pain episodes in the past that previously resolved spontaneously. Vital signs are significant for a temperature of 102.2° F (39° C). Palpation of the right subcostal area causes pain on inspiration. Abdominal ultrasound is unremarkable. What is the next best step in the diagnosis of this patient?

   - **The next best step in the diagnosis is to obtain a HIDA scan.**
   - This multiparous woman over the age of 40 years complains of right upper abdominal pain for the past 4 hours.
   - She has had similar pain episodes in the past that used to resolve spontaneously.
   - These episodes are most likely consistent with the biliary colic.
   - Vital signs are significant for a fever of 102.2° F (39° C).
   - Palpation of the right subcostal area causes pain on inspiration.
   - This phenomenon is known as Murphy's sign and is present in patients with acute cholecystitis.
   - Fever further supports the diagnosis of acute cholecystitis rather than biliary colic in this patient.
   - However, abdominal ultrasound is unremarkable.
   - If the patient is suspected to have acute cholecystitis but the ultrasound is unremarkable, the best next step in the diagnosis is HIDA scan.
   - Failure of gallbladder visualization on HIDA scan suggests the cystic duct obstruction and confirms the diagnosis of acute cholecystitis.

REVIEW QUESTIONS

2. An 18-year-old male college student is brought to the emergency department by his friend because of severe left upper quadrant pain for the past hour. The pain started when someone hit him in the abdomen while playing rugby. The patient has a past medical history notable for a sore throat and severe fatigue for the past month. Vital signs show blood pressure of 80/65 mmHg and heart rate of 135 beats/min. What is the most likely cause of this patient's current symptoms?

    - **The most likely cause of the patient's current symptoms is splenic rupture.**
    - This 18-year-old college student reports severe left upper quadrant pain for the past hour.
    - The pain started when someone hit him in the abdomen while playing rugby.
    - The left upper quadrant pain and the history of trauma raises suspicion for splenic injury.
    - Additionally, he has a past medical history of sore throat and severe fatigue for the past month, suggestive of infectious mononucleosis.
    - Infectious mononucleosis can cause splenomegaly and predispose the patient to traumatic splenic rupture.
    - Vital signs are significant for hypotension with the blood pressure of 80/65 mmHg and the tachycardia with the heart rate of 135 beats/min.
    - Hemodynamic instability with left upper quadrant pain is most consistent with splenic rupture.

3. A 65-year-old man is brought to the emergency department by his daughter because of severe upper abdominal pain radiating to the back for the past 30 minutes. He has been smoking 3 packs of cigarettes per day for the past 40 years. Vital signs are significant for a blood pressure of 85/70 mmHg and a heart rate of 136 beats/min. Physical examination shows epigastric tenderness with a pulsatile abdominal mass. What is the next best step in the diagnosis of this patient?

    - **The next best step in the diagnosis of this patient is to obtain an abdominal ultrasound asap to confirm AAA rupture.**
    - This 65-year-old man reports severe upper abdominal pain radiating to the back for the past 30 minutes.
    - He has an extensive smoking history predisposing him to vascular disease.
    - Vital signs are significant for hypotension with blood pressure of 85/70 mmHg and tachycardia with heart rate of 136 beats/min.
    - Physical examination shows epigastric tenderness with pulsatile abdominal mass suggestive of an abdominal aortic aneurysm with vitals concerning for rupture.
    - Abdominal ultrasound will confirm the AAA rupture and vascular surgery should be consulted immediately.

REVIEW QUESTIONS

4. A 7-year-old boy is brought to the emergency department by his parents because of vomiting and right lower abdominal pain for the past hour. Vital signs are significant for a temperature of 100.4° F (38° C). Extension and internal rotation of the right hip as well as palpation of the left lower quadrant all exacerbate the right lower quadrant pain. What is the best treatment option for this patient?

   - **The best treatment option for this patient is urgent appendectomy.**
   - This 7-year-old boy presents with vomiting and right lower abdominal pain for the past hour.
   - His vital signs are significant for a fever of 100.4° F (38° C).
   - Extension and internal rotation of the right hip as well as palpation of the left lower quadrant all exacerbate the right lower quadrant pain.
   - Pain exacerbation on extension of the right hip is known as psoas sign.
   - On the other hand, worsening of the pain on internal rotation of the right hip is called obturator sign.
   - If palpation in the left lower quadrant exacerbates the right lower quadrant pain, this phenomenon is known as Rovsing's sign.
   - Positive psoas sign, obturator sign, and Rovsing's sign all suggest the diagnosis of acute appendicitis.

5. A 25-year-old woman is brought to the emergency department by her mother because of vomiting and abdominal pain for the past 4 hours. Her past medical history includes laparoscopy for ruptured ectopic pregnancy 2 years ago. Vital signs include temperature of 104° F (40° C), blood pressure of 80/60 mmHg, heart rate of 155 beats/min, and respiratory rate of 16 breaths/min. Physical examination shows diffuse abdominal pain with rebound tenderness, rigidity and guarding. Serum β-hCG is undetectable. The abdominal X-ray shows dilated bowel loops and air-fluid levels along with air under the diaphragm. Intravenous fluids and antibiotics are promptly initiated. Which of the following is the next best step in the management of this patient?

   A. Pelvic ultrasound
   B. Abdominal CT scan
   C. IV metoclopramide
   D. Emergent laparotomy

- **The correct answer is option D.**
- This 25-year-old woman is brought to the emergency department because of vomiting and abdominal pain for the past 4 hours.
- Her past medical history includes laparoscopy for ruptured ectopic pregnancy 2 years ago which predisposes her to abdominal adhesions and bowel obstruction.
- Vital signs indicate she is febrile and hemodynamically unstable.
- Physical examination shows diffuse abdominal pain with rebound tenderness, rigidity and guarding. These findings are consistent with an acute abdomen and peritonitis.
- The abdominal X-ray shows dilated bowel loops and air-fluid levels along with air under the diaphragm, indicating small bowel obstruction complicated by bowel rupture and pneumoperitoneum.
- The next best step in the management of a hemodynamically unstable patient with an acute abdomen is emergent laparotomy.
- Option A is incorrect. Although this patient is at risk of ectopic pregnancy based on her past history, serum beta-hCG is undetectable making this diagnosis unlikely. Plus, the patient is hemodynamically unstable and requires emergent intervention without wasting time.
- Option B is incorrect because abdominal CT scan will not change the management of this patient. She will still require laparotomy so performing CT scan in this particular case would be a waste of time.
- Option C is incorrect. Although this patient needs antiemetic for vomiting, metoclopramide is contraindicated in patients with bowel obstruction. This is because metoclopramide increases GI motility and exacerbates the symptoms of bowel obstruction.

Burn Degree	Tissue Involvement	Clinical Features
First degree (superficial)	- Epidermis	- Resembles a sunburn: localized, tender, blanching erythema - No blisters - Intact capillary refill
Second degree (partial thickness)	- Epidermis and parts of dermis	- Tender, edematous, mottled, skin - Blisters present
Third degree (full thickness)	- Epidermis and all of dermis	- Painless, white, charred, leathery areas of skin - No blanching
Fourth degree	- Epidermis, dermis, and all underlying tissue (e.g. adipose, muscle, bone)	- Painless, white, charred, leathery areas of skin - No blanching - Disfiguring

TABLE 14.1.3 - Thermal Burns

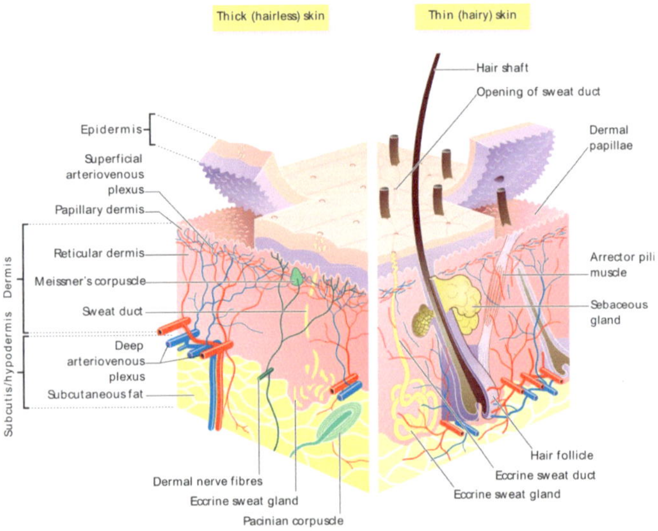

FIGURE 14.1.36 - Layers of Skin

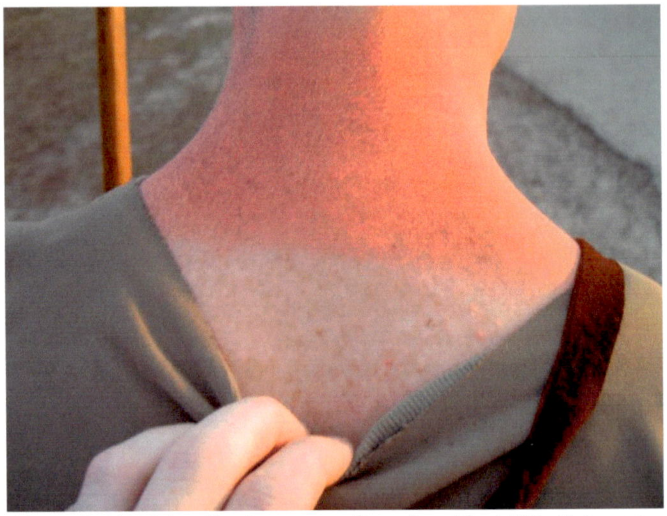

FIGURE 14.1.37 - First Degree Burn

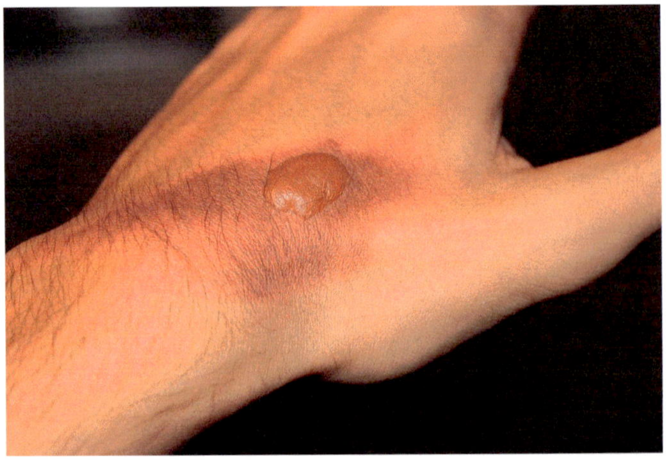

FIGURE 14.1.38 - Second Degree Burn

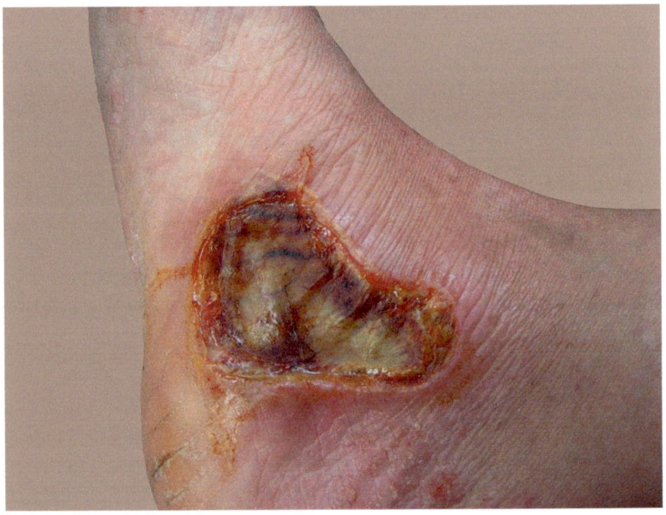

FIGURE 14.1.39 - Third Degree Burn

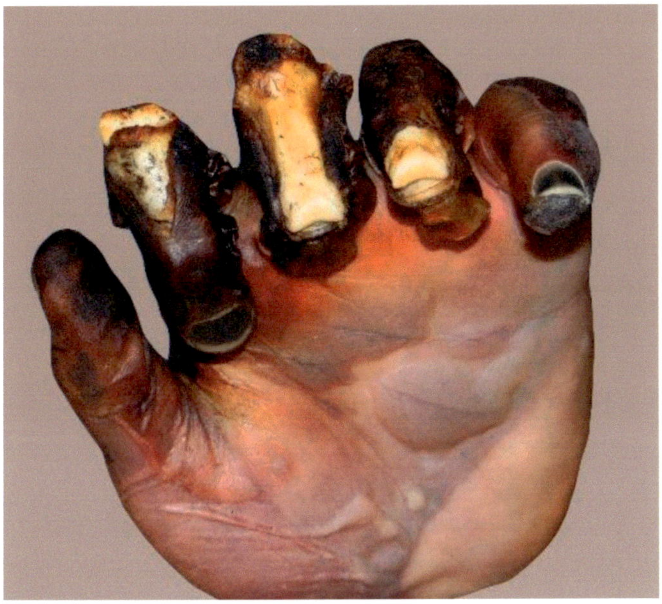

goga312 at Russian Wikipedia, CC BY-SA 3.0 <https://creativecommons.org/licenses/by-sa/3.0>, via Wikimedia Commons

FIGURE 14.1.40 - Fourth Degree Burn

I. Chemical Burns
  A. Alkali burns
    1. More damaging and lead to coagulation necrosis
  B. Acid burns
    1. Lead to liquefactive necrosis
  C. Treatment
    1. Decontamination and irrigation
    2. Transferral to burn center

II. Electrical Burns
  A. Examples: lightning strikes, electrical outlets
  B. Acute complications
    1. Cardiac arrhythmias (e.g. asystole, ventricular fibrillation)
    2. Muscle necrosis and myoglobinuria
    3. Renal failure
  C. Chronic complication: cataracts
  D. Treatment: monitor for arrhythmias, transfer to a burn center

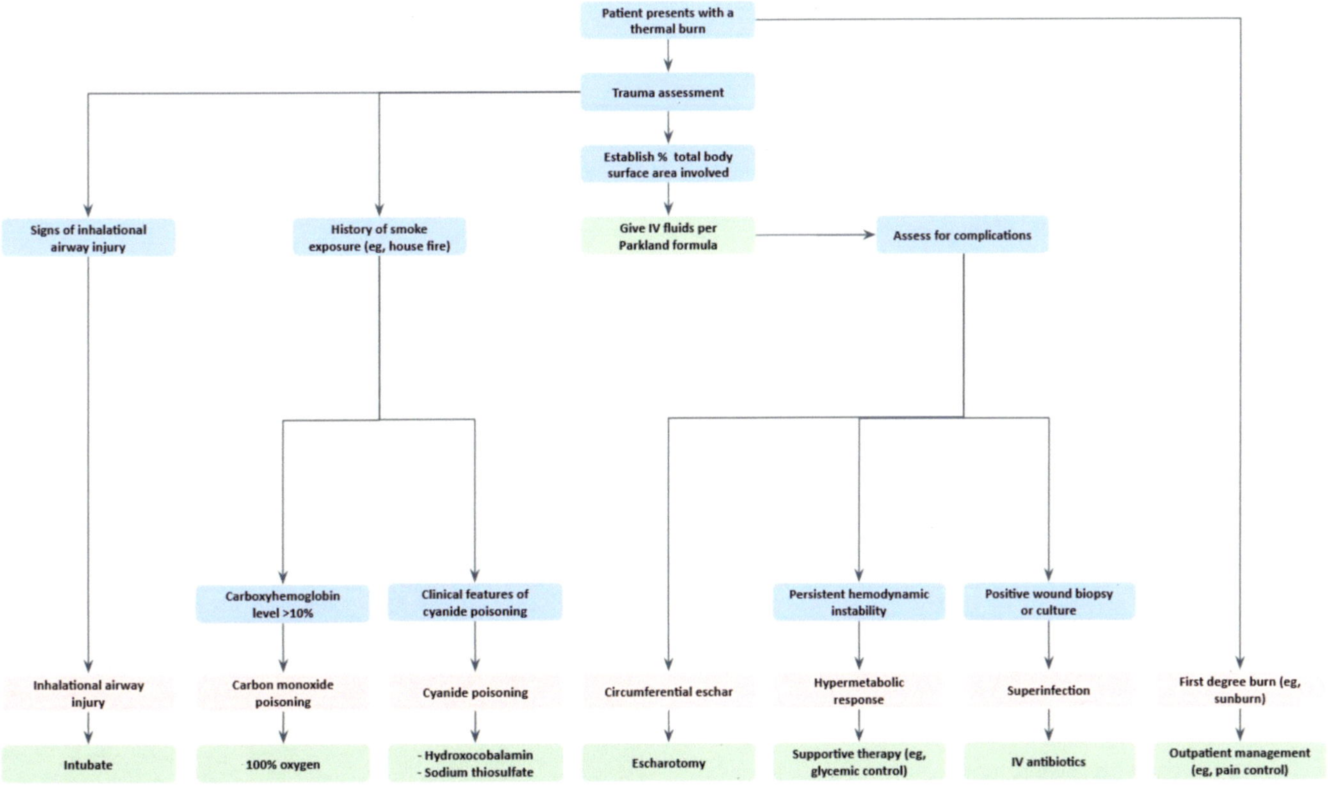

FIGURE 14.1.41 - Approach to Burn Injuries in the Emergency Department

Findings Suggestive of Inhalational Airway Injury
- Carbonaceous sputum
- Signs of oropharyngeal inflammation (e.g. pharyngeal erythema)
- Facial burns
- Singed eyebrows or nasal hairs
- Change in voice quality (e.g. stridor)

TABLE 14.1.4 - Features of Inhalational Airway Injury

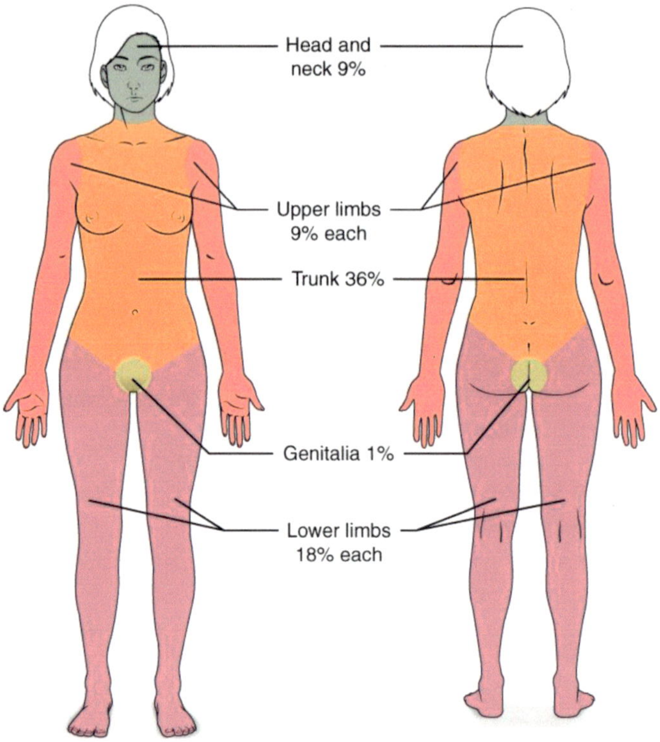

FIGURE 14.1.42 - Rule of 9s

III. Parkland Formula
  A. Used to manage patients with second or third degree burns covering > 20% of their total body surface area (TBSA)
  B. Estimates total fluid needs within the first 24 hours per the equation:
    1. Total fluid requirement = TBSA (%) x weight (kg) x 4 cc/kg
    2. Give half of fluid requirements within first 8 hours
    3. Give second half within the next 16 hours
  C. Titrate intravenous fluids to achieve adequate urine output

IV. Circumferential Eschar
  A. A full-thickness (third degree) circumferential burn that disrupts venous and lymphatic drainage
  B. Increases risk for acute compartment syndrome distal to the burn
    1. Treat with escharotomy

V. Hypermetabolic Response to Burn Injury
  A. Moderate-to-severe burn injuries lead to release of inflammatory mediators and stress hormones (e.g. catecholamines, cortisol)
  B. Clinical features
    1. Tachycardia, hypertension, hyperthermia
    2. Hyperglycemia (due to insulin resistance)
    3. Increased tissue catabolism (e.g. muscle wasting)
  C. Diagnosis is clinical
  D. Address the underlying burn injury (e.g. early burn excision)
  E. Offer supportive therapy
    1. Beta blockers to control blood pressure and heart rate
    2. Insulin to control hyperglycemia
    3. Nutritional support to offset increased catabolism

VI. Superinfection
  A. Superinfection of a burn injury should be suspected when
    1. A second degree burn progresses to a third degree burn during inpatient stay
    2. There is green pigment around the burn wound
    3. There is black necrotic skin around the burn wound
  B. Most common pathogens: *Pseudomonas aeruginosa* and gram-positive cocci (e.g. *Staphylococcus aureus*)
  C. Diagnosis
    1. Positive wound culture
    2. Punch biopsy with > 100,000 bacteria/gram of burned tissue
  D. Treatment: IV antibiotics (e.g. aminoglycosides, vancomycin)
  E. Complication: burn wound sepsis

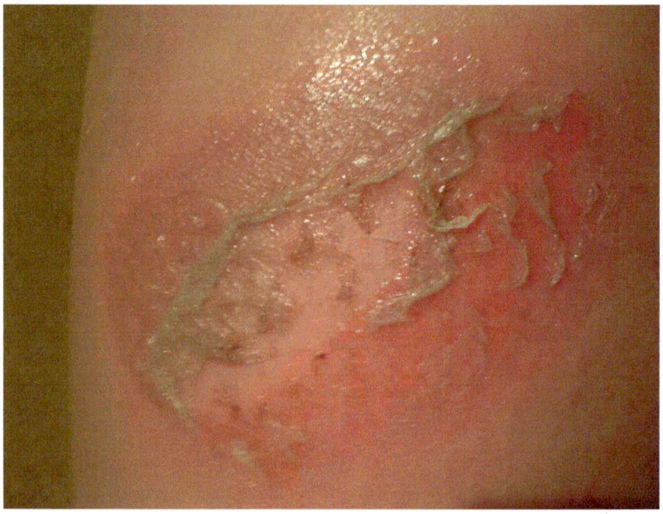

FIGURE 14.1.43 - Burn Wound Infection

VII. Burn Wound Sepsis
   A. Burn wound sepsis diagnostic criteria
      1. Temperature < 36.5° C (97.7° F) or > 39° C (102.2° F)
      2. Systolic blood pressure < 90 mmHg, despite resuscitation
      3. Heart rate > 90 beats per minute
      4. Respiratory rate > 30 breaths per minute
   B. Treatment: broad-spectrum IV antibiotics (e.g. piperacillin/tazobactam)
      1. Consider coverage against MRSA (e.g. vancomycin)

VIII. Burn Injury Management Pearls
   A. Lactated ringers is the IV fluid of choice for burn patients
      1. Normal saline increases risk for hyperchloremic metabolic acidosis
   B. Prophylactic topical antimicrobials (e.g. silver sulfadiazine) can be useful
      1. No benefit of using oral or intravenous antibiotics prophylactically
   C. Consider stress (Curling) ulcer prophylaxis (e.g. PPIs, H2-blockers)
   D. Consider tetanus vaccination

Indications to Transfer Patients to the Burn Center
- Inhalational injury
- Electrical or chemical burns
- Burns affecting face, hands, feet, or perineum
- Second degree burns affecting > 10% of total body surface area
- Third degree burns
- Suspected child abuse

TABLE 14.1.5 - Indications to Transfer Patients to the Burn Center

REVIEW QUESTIONS

1. What is the degree of burn injury to this patient's palm?

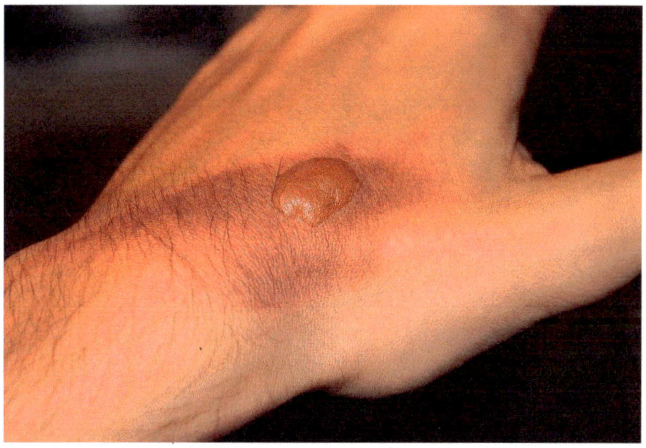

- **This patient's palm injury is a second degree burn.**
- It is a second degree burn because of the notable blisters.
- First degree burns do not exhibit blisters, and third or fourth degree burns tend to appear either extensively charred or white and leathery, which isn't the case on this patient's palm.
- The clinician could ask the patient if the palmar lesion is painful or not. Presence of pain would be consistent with a second degree burn, whereas absence of pain would be more consistent with a third degree burn.

REVIEW QUESTIONS

2. A 25-year-old patient is brought to the emergency department by his friend with second and third degree burns covering the back of his head and neck, his entire back, and the posterior aspect of his left leg. His weight is 143 lbs. What is the minimum amount of fluid that this patient should be given in the first 24 hours?

- **The minimum amount of fluid that this patient should be given is 8 liters in the first 24 hours.**
- The first step is to calculate the percent of the total body surface area affected by the burns. The "back of his head and neck" equates to 4.5%, "his entire back" equates to 18%, and "the posterior aspect of his left leg" equates to 9%.
- In sum, 31.5% of this patient's total body surface area has been injured by burns.
- The next step is to use this number along with his weight in kilograms in the Parkland formula. Calculations show 8,190 cc or 8,190 mL of fluid, which means that this patient should receive roughly 8 liters of fluid in the first 24 hours.
- Per the Parkland formula, half of this fluid should be given in the first 8 hours and the other half should be given over the next 16 hours. Therefore, the patient should receive about 4 L or 4000 mL of fluid in the first 8 hours, which means that the patient will need to receive 500 mL of fluid per hour in the first 8 hours.
- The remaining 4 L of fluid should then be given over the next 16 hours, which means a rate of 250 mL of fluid per hour.

3. What are the clinical features that should prompt suspicion of compartment syndrome of an extremity?

- **Clinical features that should prompt suspicion of compartment syndrome of an extremity are pain, paresthesias, pallor, pulselessness, poikilothermia, and paralysis.**
- The clinical features of compartment syndrome can be remembered with the mnemonic of "Six Ps": pain, especially on passive stretching of the extremity, paresthesias, pallor, pulselessness, poikilothermia, and paralysis.
- Pain and paresthesias are the earliest findings of compartment syndrome, and these symptoms should be taken very seriously in patients with circumferential eschars.

4. What is the primary way of distinguishing burn wound sepsis from hypermetabolic response to burn injury?

- **The key difference is that burn wound sepsis requires a confirmed burn wound superinfection for diagnosis. In other words, patients must either have a positive culture or a positive wound biopsy.**
- **Hypermetabolic response to burn injury, on the other hand, will cause refractory hemodynamic instability in the setting of negative cultures or biopsy results.**
- Both of these complications of burn injuries can present with refractory hemodynamic instability.

REVIEW QUESTIONS

5. A 27-year-old man is rescued from a burning apartment complex and brought to the emergency department via ambulance with extensive burns. He is unresponsive and vitals show temperature of 97.2° F (36.2° C), blood pressure of 87/55 mmHg, pulse of 110 beats per minute, and respiratory rate of 21 breaths per minute. Physical examination shows burns on his face and oropharyngeal erythema. There are partial-thickness and full-thickness burns on his back, abdomen, and lower extremities. The resident pages the burn unit in anticipation of transferring the patient to their care following initial stabilization. Which of the following is the next best in management while the patient is in the emergency department?

    A. Normal saline infusion
    B. Beta blockers
    C. Intravenous antibiotics
    D. Endotracheal intubation

- **The correct answer is option D.**
- This patient presents to the emergency department with extensive thermal burns.
- He is hemodynamically unstable and physical examination reveals extensive burn injuries. Importantly, he has burns on his face along with oropharyngeal erythema.
- Signs of oropharyngeal inflammation and facial burns are findings that are strongly suggestive of inhalational airway injury.
- Additionally, during the trauma assessment of a patient with thermal burn injuries, identification of signs of inhalational airway injury should prompt urgent intubation because these patients are at high risk of developing airway edema and subsequent obstruction. This is why endotracheal intubation is the correct answer.
- Option A is incorrect because normal saline infusion is critical to first secure this patient's airway because of the high risk of airway edema and compromise in patients with inhalational airway injury.
- Additionally, the fluid of choice in burn patients is lactated ringers, not normal saline. This is because normal saline can cause hyperchloremic metabolic acidosis when given in high amounts because of its supraphysiologic chloride concentration. Lactated ringers is a more balanced fluid that does not increase patients' risk for developing a metabolic acidosis.
- Option B is incorrect because beta blockers will likely be detrimental in this patient because he is quite hypotensive and is likely volume depleted.
- Option C is incorrect because intravenous or oral antibiotics are not useful in prophylaxis against burn wound superinfections; only topical antimicrobial agents are.

I. Hypothermia: Definition
   A. Mild hypothermia (32 - 35° C or 89.6 - 95° F)
   B. Moderate hypothermia (28 - 32° C or 82.4 - 89.6° F)
   C. Severe hypothermia (< 28° C or < 82.4° F)

II. Hypothermia: Pathophysiology
   A. Increased heat loss (e.g. cold environment)
   B. Decreased heat production (e.g. hypothyroidism)
   C. Disrupted circulation (e.g. diabetics, smokers)
   D. Thermal dysregulation (e.g. stroke)

III. Hypothermia: Risk Factors
   A. Extremes of age (e.g. elderly, infants)
   B. Alcoholics
   C. Anorexia nervosa
   D. Hypothyroidism
   E. Drugs (e.g. opioids)
   F. Sepsis
   G. Spinal cord injuries

IV. Hypothermia: Clinical Features
   A. Mild hypothermia (32 - 35° C or 89.6 - 95° F)
      1. Shivering, tachycardia, ataxia, cold-induced diuresis
   B. Moderate hypothermia (28 - 32° C or 82.4 - 89.6° F)
      1. Altered mental status, no shivering
      2. Arrhythmias (e.g. pulseless electrical activity, atrial fibrillation)
   C. Severe hypothermia (< 28° C or < 82.4° F)
      1. Arrhythmias, coma, hypotension,

V. Hypothermia: Diagnosis
   A. Direct core temperature measurement
   B. Look for etiology (e.g. hypothyroidism, drugs)
   C. Hyperglycemia
   D. Hyperkalemia
   E. Acidosis
      1. Respiratory
      2. Metabolic
   F. Coagulopathy
   G. ECG may reveal a J wave (Osborn wave)

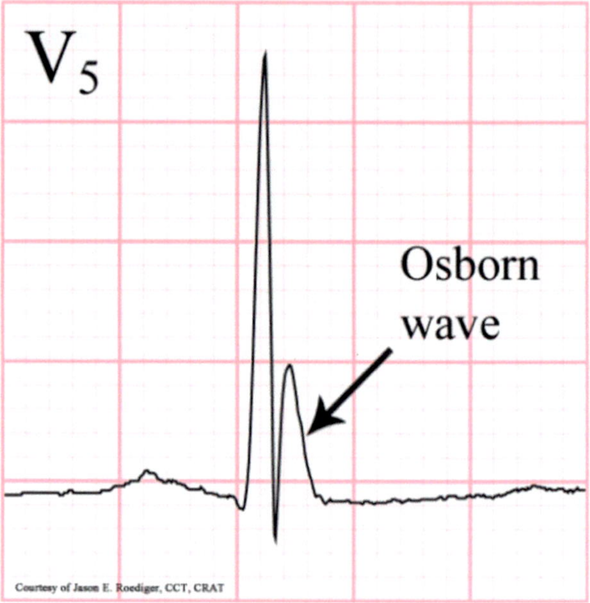

FIGURE 14.1.44 - ECG: J Wave (Osborn Wave)

VI. Hypothermia: Management
   A. General measures
      1. Place the patient in a warm environment
      2. Remove cold/wet clothing
      3. Supportive therapy (e.g. warm crystalloid fluids and electrolytes)
      4. Monitor for arrhythmias (e.g. bradycardia)
   B. Initiate rewarming protocols based on severity of hypothermia
   C. Mild hypothermia (< 35° C or < 95° F) is treated with passive external rewarming
      1. Remove wet clothing
      2. Insulate patient with blankets
   D. Moderate hypothermia (< 32° C or < 89.6° F) is treated with active external rewarming
      1. Warm blankets
      2. Warm water bath
      3. Forced-air warming system (e.g. Bair Hugger)
   E. Severe hypothermia (< 28° C or < 82.4° F) is treated with active internal rewarming
      1. Warm IV fluids
      2. Warm peritoneal lavage
      3. Extracorporeal rewarming (e.g. hemodialysis)
   F. Endotracheal intubation for comatose patients
   G. Frostbite (frozen skin tissue)
      1. Rapid rewarming in a warm water bath (37-39° C or 98.6-102.2° F)
      2. Pain medications
      3. Wound care, assessment for debridement
      4. Thrombolysis if tissue is necrotic and at risk for amputation
   H. Rewarming with hot air is not recommended
   I. Management of the core temperature takes precedence

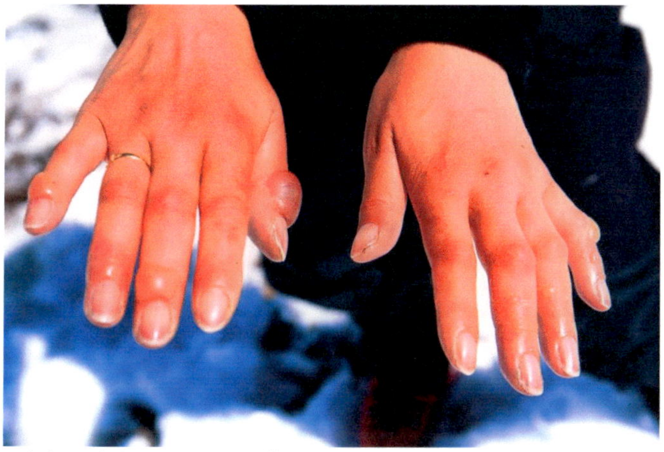

FIGURE 14.1.45 - Frostbite Injury

VII. Hyperthermia: Definition
   A. Elevation of core body temperature above 40° C or 104° F due to failure of thermoregulation
   B. Not synonymous with fever

VIII. Hyperthermia: Risk Factors
   A. Extremes of age (e.g. infants, elderly)
   B. Physical labor in a hot, humid environment
      1. Athletes
      2. Military recruits
   C. Obesity
   D. Sepsis
   E. Drugs (e.g. MDMA, diphenhydramine, antipsychotics)

IX. Hyperthermia: Clinical Features
   A. Heat fatigue (e.g. heavy sweating, tiredness)
   B. Heat exhaustion
      1. Cool, clammy skin
      2. Headaches, dizziness, fainting
      3. Muscle cramps
      4. Increased risk for heat stroke
   C. Heat stroke

X. Hyperthermia: Diagnosis
   A. Direct core temperature measurement
   B. Consider special cases of hyperthermia:
      1. Malignant hyperthermia in the postoperative period
      2. Neuroleptic malignant syndrome in a patient on antipsychotics
      3. Serotonin syndrome in a patient on serotonergic medications

XI. Hyperthermia: Management
   A. General measures
      1. Active cooling with cold water, wet blankets, ice, or fans
   B. Consider benzodiazepines or phenothiazines to stop shivering
   C. Antipyretics are not useful in treatment of hyperthermia

	Malignant Hyperthermia	Neuroleptic Malignant Syndrome	Serotonin Syndrome
Definition	- Hypermetabolic reaction to particular drugs, often presenting as postoperative fever	- Adverse reaction to antipsychotic medications	- Adverse reaction to excessive serotonin levels in the system
Pathophysiology	- Defect of RyR receptors on sarcoplasmic reticulum	- Dopaminergic blockade	- Overactivation of serotonergic pathways
Risk factors	- Anesthesia (e.g. halothane, succinylcholine)	- Antipsychotic medications (e.g. haloperidol, risperidone)	- Serotonin-related medications (e.g. SSRIs, TCAs)
Clinical features	- Hyperthermia - Altered mental status - Muscle rigidity	- Hyperthermia - Altered mental status - Autonomic instability - Muscle rigidity - Myoglobinuria - Elevated muscle enzymes (e.g. CK)	- Hyperthermia - Autonomic instability - Agitation - Neuromuscular hyperactivity (e.g. clonus, hyperreflexia)
Diagnosis	- Clinical diagnosis	- Clinical diagnosis	- Clinical diagnosis
Management	- Stop anesthesia - Dantrolene	- Stop antipsychotics - Dantrolete or bromocriptine	- Stop serotonin-related medications - Cyproheptadine

TABLE 14.1.6 - Causes of Hyperthermia

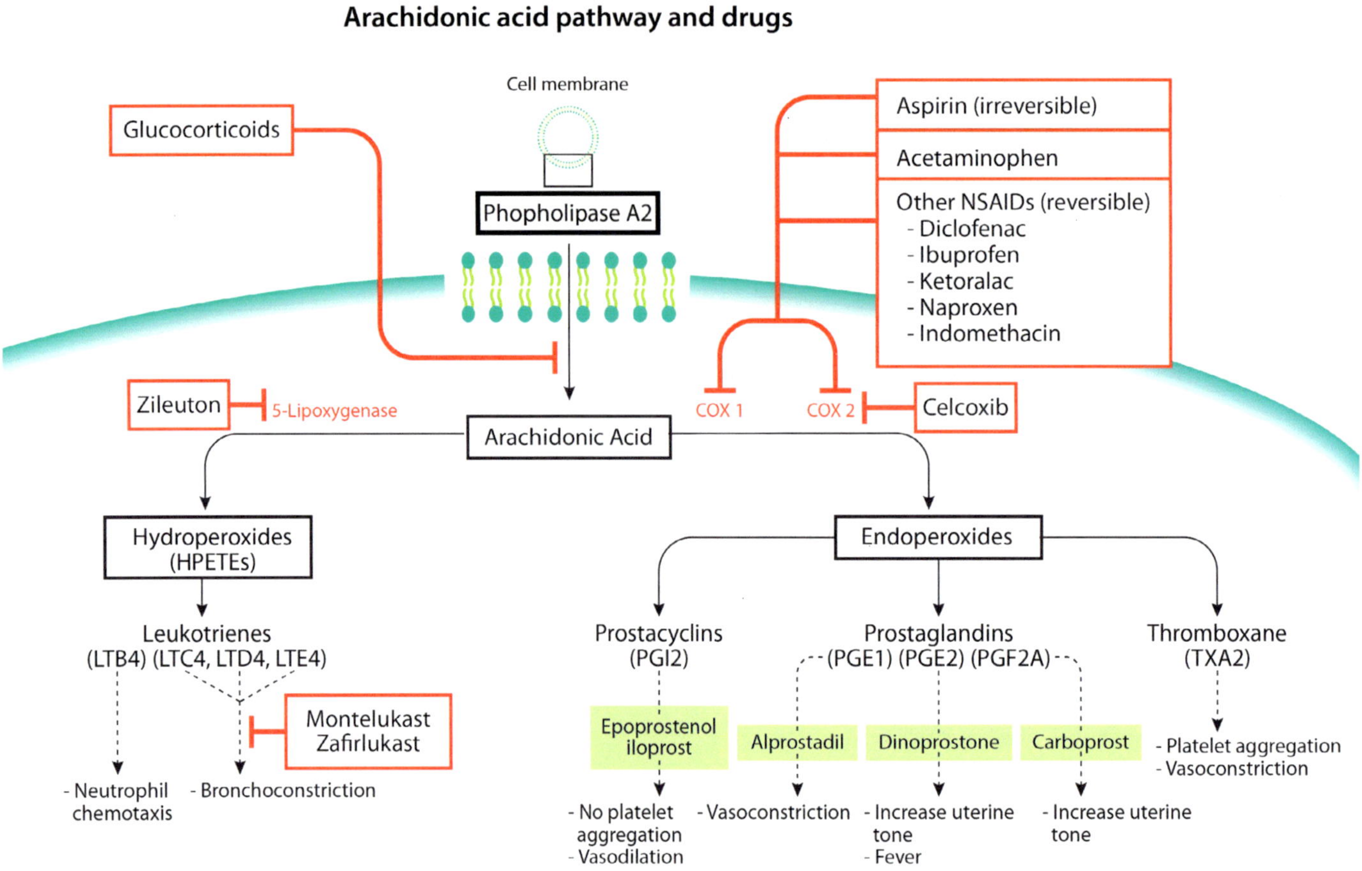

FIGURE 14.1.46 - Arachidonic Acid Pathway

XII. Heat Stroke: Definition
- A. Core body temperature > 40° C or > 104° F with central nervous system dysfunction (e.g. altered mental status)
  1. Nonexertional heat stroke
  2. Exertional heat stroke
- B. Life-threatening disorder

XIII. Heat Stroke: Pathophysiology
- A. Nonexertional heat stroke
  1. Impaired thermoregulation
     a. Exertional heat stroke
- B. Insufficient dissipation of heat during strenuous physical activity

XIV. Heat Stroke: Risk Factors
- A. Nonexertional heat stroke
  1. Elderly patients with chronic medical conditions (e.g. cardiovascular disease, physical disability)
- B. Exertional heat stroke
  1. Athletes (e.g. marathon runners)
  2. Military recruits (e.g. bootcamp training)
  3. Strenuous physical activity in hot, humid environments

XV. Heat Stroke: Clinical Features
- A. Central nervous system dysfunction (e.g. altered mental status)
- B. Hemodynamic instability (e.g. hypotension, tachycardia)
- C. End-organ dysfunction
  1. Acute respiratory distress syndrome (ARDS)
  2. Hepatic failure, renal failure
  3. Disseminated intravascular coagulation
- D. Rhabdomyolysis

XVI. Heat Stroke: Diagnosis
- A. Clinical diagnosis
- B. Rule out other causes of hyperthermia in the setting of central nervous system dysfunction (e.g. malignant hyperthermia, thyroid storm)

XVII. Heat Stroke: Management
- A. Address airway, breathing, circulation
- B. Initiate rapid cooling
  1. Ice water immersion for most patients
  2. Evaporative cooling for elderly with nonexertional heat strokes
- C. Offer supportive therapy (e.g. replete fluids and electrolytes)
- D. Treat complications (e.g. mechanical ventilation for ARDS)
- E. Antipyretics are not useful

REVIEW QUESTIONS

1. A 23-year-old man is brought to the emergency department by helicopter after a snowmobiling accident. His core body temperature on admission is 87.8° F (31° C). What is the best next step in management?
   - **The best next step in management is active external rewarming.**
   - The patient's core temperature of 87.8° F (31° C), consistent with a diagnosis of moderate hypothermia.
   - In addition to the general measures, such as removing wet or cold clothing, the best treatment for moderate hypothermia is active external rewarming, which may include interventions like warm blankets, a warm water bath, or a forced-air warming system.
2. A 40-year-old woman undergoing elective cholecystectomy suddenly develops a high fever and muscle rigidity immediately following anesthesia. What is the next best step in management?
   - **The next best step in management is to stop anesthesia and provide active cooling and dantrolene.**
   - High fever and muscle rigidity immediately following anesthesia is most likely malignant hyperthermia.
   - Hence, the next best step in management is to stop the anesthesia and treat the patient with active cooling and dantrolene.
   - Notably, halothane and succinylcholine are the two anesthetic agents that are most commonly associated with the development of malignant hyperthermia in predisposed individuals.
3. What is the key clinical feature that distinguishes hyperthermia from heat stroke?
   - **The key distinguishing feature is that heat stroke also presents with central nervous system dysfunction.**
   - Hyperthermia is defined as an elevation in core body temperature above 40° C or 104° F due to failure of thermoregulation.
   - Heat stroke, on the other hand, is defined as an elevation of core body temperature above 40° C or 104° F and central nervous system dysfunction, such as confusion.
4. A 52-year-old man is brought to the emergency department in July after he collapsed in his backyard. He is accompanied by his wife who says that they were doing yard work when the patient suddenly became confused and collapsed shortly thereafter. He has a history of hypertension, coronary artery disease, depression, and insomnia. He takes lisinopril, aspirin, atorvastatin, sertraline, risperidone, and trazodone. Vital signs show blood pressure of 110/70 mmHg, pulse of 94 beats per minute, and temperature of 105.8° F (41° C). He is still confused but responds to commands. On physical examination, his skin is warm and dry. Pulmonary, cardiovascular, and abdominal aspects of the examination are unremarkable. Muscle tone is within normal limits throughout, and deep tendon reflexes are normal. Which of the following is the most likely diagnosis?

   A. Malignant hyperthermia
   B. Heat stroke
   C. Neuroleptic malignant syndrome
   D. Serotonin syndrome

   - **The correct answer is option B.**
   - This older gentleman collapsed doing yard work on a hot summer day in July.
   - On admission, the patient had a temperature of 105.8° F (41° C) and was confused. This prompts suspicion of heat stroke.
   - This diagnosis is further supported by the fact that he has a known history of coronary artery disease and that he takes risperidone, which has anticholinergic side effects and can therefore predispose to or exacerbate hyperthermia.
   - Option A is incorrect because patients with malignant hyperthermia exhibit generalized muscle rigidity, which isn't the case in this patient, as his muscle tone was within normal limits throughout.
   - Option C is incorrect because neuroleptic malignant syndrome also typically involves generalized muscle rigidity, which is not the case in this patient, making this diagnosis less likely.
   - Option D is incorrect because patients with serotonin syndrome typically exhibit clonus and hyperreflexia, which is not the case in this patient, as his reflexes were normal and symmetric.

I. Anticholinergic Poisoning: Definition
   A. Chemical substance inhibits the binding of acetylcholine to its receptor

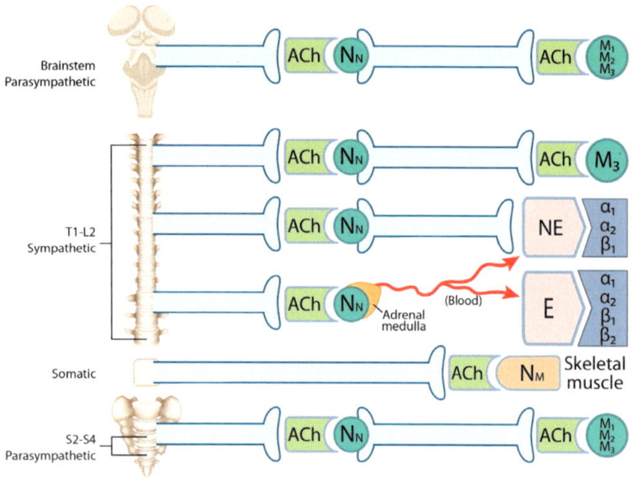

FIGURE 14.1.47 - Receptors of Autonomic Nervous System

II. Anticholinergic Poisoning: Pathophysiology
   A. Acetylcholine binding to muscarinic receptors causes a parasympathetic response (rest and digest)
   B. Inhibiting this process via poisoning causes an exaggerated sympathetic response
   C. Anticholinergic substances inhibit the muscarinic receptors
   D. No effect on nicotinic receptors
      1. No effect on the muscles

Anticholinergic Substance	Examples
Antimuscarinic drugs	- Atropine - Scopolamine
First-generation antihistamines	- Diphenhydramine - Cyproheptadine
Tricyclic antidepressants	- Amitriptyline - Imipramine
Antipsychotics	- Chlorpromazine - Clozapine
Inhaled bronchodilators	- Ipratropium - Tiotropium
Overactive bladder medications	- Oxybutynin - Tolterodine
Parkinson's disease medications	- Trihexyphenidyl - Benztropine
Plants	- Jimson weed - Deadly nightshade

TABLE 14.1.7 - Anticholinergic Substances

III. Anticholinergic Poisoning: Clinical Features
   A. "Red as a beet": inability to sweat → vasodilation to dissipate heat
   B. "Dry as a bone": decreased sweating and mucous secretions
   C. "Hot as a hare": inability to sweat causes hyperthermia
   D. "Blind as a bat": inability to accommodate causes blurry vision
   E. "Mad as a hatter": anxiety, agitation, visual hallucinations
   F. "Full as a flask": urinary retention and constipation
   G. "Fast as a fiddle": inhibition of vagus nerve → unopposed tachycardia

IV. Anticholinergic Poisoning: Diagnosis
   A. Clinical diagnosis
      1. If physostigmine reduces the symptoms, this supports the diagnosis

V. Anticholinergic Poisoning: Management
   A. Supportive therapy
      1. Stabilize airway, breathing, circulation
      2. Cardiac monitoring and pulse oximetry
   B. Physostigmine (acetylcholinesterase inhibitor)

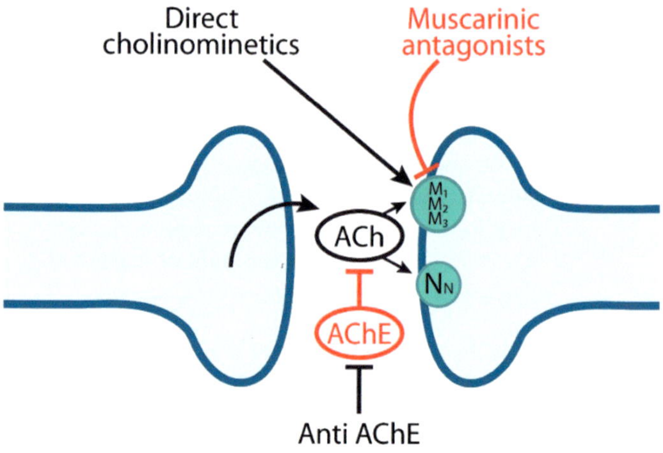

FIGURE 14.1.48 - Mechanism of Action of Physostigmine (Anticholinesterase Inhibitor)

VI. Acetylcholinesterase Inhibitor Poisoning: Definition
   A. Poisoning with an agent that inhibits acetylcholinesterase - an enzyme that breaks down acetylcholine

VII. Acetylcholinesterase Inhibitor Poisoning: Pathophysiology
   A. Acetylcholine builds up at muscarinic and nicotinic receptors
      1. Since nicotinic receptors are affected, skeletal muscles are affected

VIII. Acetylcholinesterase Inhibitor Poisoning: Etiology
- A. Pesticides
  1. Contain organophosphates
  2. Absorbed through skin, lungs, and gastrointestinal tract
- B. Acetylcholinesterase inhibitor medications
  1. Pyridostigmine (Myasthenia gravis)
  2. Donepezil (Alzheimer dementia)

IX. Acetylcholinesterase Inhibitor Poisoning: Clinical Features
- A. Autonomic nervous system
  1. Exaggerated parasympathetic response
  2. Remembered by the mnemonic “SLUDGE/BBB”
     - **a)** **S**alivation
     - **b)** **L**acrimation
     - **c)** **U**rination
     - **d)** **D**efecation
     - **e)** **G**astric **E**mesis
     - **f)** **B**ronchorrhea
     - **g)** **B**ronchospasm
     - **h)** **B**radycardia
- B. Effects on skeletal muscles
  1. Fasciculations
  2. Muscle weakness
  3. Paralysis

X. Acetylcholinesterase Inhibitor Poisoning: Diagnosis
- A. Clinical diagnosis
- B. Measure RBC acetylcholinesterase activity
- C. Diagnosis is supported if a trial of atropine reduces symptoms
  1. Atropine inhibits acetylcholine from binding to its receptor

XI. Acetylcholinesterase Inhibitor Poisoning: Treatment
- A. Decontamination
- B. Supportive therapy (e.g. intubation, IV fluids)
- C. Avoid succinylcholine when intubating
  1. Metabolized by acetylcholinesterase
  2. May cause prolonged neuromuscular blockade
- D. Atropine + pralidoxime
  1. Atropine inhibits muscarinic receptors
  2. Pralidoxime reactivates acetylcholinesterase at muscarinic and nicotinic receptors
- E. Always administer atropine before pralidoxime
  1. Pralidoxime transiently inhibits acetylcholinesterase when administered
  2. Initially causes more ACh buildup and worsens symptoms

Condition	Etiology	Key Features
Anticholinergic toxicity	- Medications (antihistamines, antipsychotics, TCAs), - Plants (Jimson Weed, Deadly Nightshade)	- “Red as a Beet,” “ Dry as a Bone,” “Hot as a Hare,” “Blind as a Bat,” “Mad as a Hatter,” “Full as a Flask,” “Fast as a Fiddle” - No effect on skeletal muscle - Treat with physostigmine
Acetylcholinesterase inhibitor poisoning	- Pesticides containing organophosphates - Physostigmine, neostigmine, edrophonium, donepezil	- CNS depression - “SLUDGE/BBB” - Muscular weakness, fasciculations, paralysis - Treat with atropine followed by pralidoxime

TABLE 14.1.8 - Anticholinergic Toxicity and Acetylcholinesterase Inhibitor Poisoning

REVIEW QUESTIONS

1. A 37-year-old woman is brought to the emergency department by her boyfriend due to hallucinations and confusion for the past 24 hours. Her boyfriend found an empty bottle of pills next to her. She has a history of peptic ulcer disease and schizoaffective disorder. Her medications include omeprazole, chlorpromazine, lorazepam, and sertraline. Physical examination shows flushed skin and mydriasis. Overdose of which medication most likely accounts for this patient's current symptoms?
   - **Overdose of chlorpromazine most likely accounts for this patient's current symptoms.**
   - This patient presents with hallucinations, confusion, flushing, and mydriasis after a possible suicide attempt.
   - Altered mental status, along with these physical signs, are consistent with anticholinergic toxicity.
   - The only medication from the patient's list that has anticholinergic properties is chlorpromazine. Therefore, chlorpromazine overdose most likely accounts for her current symptoms.

2. An 89-year-old woman is brought to the emergency department by her daughter because of confusion for the past 12 hours. She took scopolamine before a boat trip for motion sickness earlier in the day. Vital signs include a temperature of 102.2° F (39° C) and a heart rate of 120 beats/min. Physical examination shows flushed skin. After initial resuscitation, which medication can definitively reverse her symptoms?
   - **The medication that can definitively reverse her symptoms is physostigmine.**
   - This elderly woman presents with acute-onset confusion.
   - She presents with hyperthermia, tachycardia, and flushed skin.
   - Scopolamine, which she took before a boat trip, is an anticholinergic agent used to treat motion sickness.
   - Therefore, this patient likely has anticholinergic toxicity.
   - The medication that can definitively reverse her symptoms is physostigmine. This is an acetylcholinesterase inhibitor with high blood-brain barrier permeability. Therefore, it increases the acetylcholine levels in the synaptic clefts. Acetylcholine then displaces the anticholinergic medication from the muscarinic and nicotinic receptors reversing the patient's symptoms.

3. A 79-year-old woman with Alzheimer's dementia is brought to the emergency department by her daughter because of shortness of breath, vomiting, and excessive drooling for the last 3 hours. Her medications include donepezil and memantine. On physical examination, her pants are soiled. Vital signs include a heart rate of 40 beats/min. The patient is promptly treated with an antidote. Which test can support the diagnosis of this patient's condition?
   - **The test that can best support the diagnosis of this patient's condition is RBC acetylcholinesterase activity.**
   - This elderly woman is brought to the emergency department because of shortness of breath, vomiting, and excessive drooling.
   - On physical examination, she has soiled herself.
   - Her vital signs include a heart rate of 50 beats/min.
   - Hypersecretion and bradycardia suggest poisoning with an acetylcholinesterase inhibitor.
   - This patient takes donepezil, an acetylcholinesterase inhibitor.
   - Acetylcholinesterase inhibitor poisoning is a clinical diagnosis and does not typically require further diagnostic investigation. However, one can measure RBC acetylcholinesterase activity in order to support the diagnosis of this patient's condition.

REVIEW QUESTIONS

4. A 57-year-old man who works as a farmer is brought to the emergency department by his wife because of shortness of breath for the last hour. He was working in the fields when he suddenly felt short of breath. He vomited twice on his way to the hospital. On physical examination, he is sweating profusely, and he has soiled himself. Vital signs include a heart rate of 53 beats/min. Atropine is given, followed by pralidoxime. What is the most likely rationale for administering atropine before pralidoxime?

- **The rationale for administering atropine before pralidoxime is that atropine counteracts the transient acetylcholinesterase inhibitor effects of pralidoxime.**
- This farmer is brought to the emergency department because of shortness of breath, vomiting, and sweating,
- He has bradycardia.
- The signs of hypersecretion, along with bradycardia, suggest acetylcholinesterase inhibitor poisoning.
- Given his occupation, this patient likely is suffering from organophosphate poisoning.
- Atropine is given, followed by pralidoxime.
- The reason for this specific sequence is that pralidoxime initially causes a transient inhibition of acetylcholinesterase. Therefore, acetylcholine builds up in the synaptic cleft and worsens the symptoms. Since atropine blocks the muscarinic receptors, it will counteract the transient acetylcholinesterase inhibitor effects of pralidoxime at the muscarinic sites.

5. A 55-year-old woman is brought to the emergency department by her husband because of vomiting and diarrhea for the past 5 hours. She has a history of chronic alcoholism and medically treated myasthenia gravis. She has been admitted for methanol and ethylene glycol poisoning 7 and 10 years ago, respectively. This morning, the patient took twice the dose of her myasthenia gravis medication due to excessive weakness. Her vital signs include a temperature of 98.6° F (37° C), blood pressure of 110/80 mmHg, and heart rate of 49 beats/min. Physical examination shows miosis, excessive salivation, and bilateral wheezing. The laboratory studies are unremarkable. Which of the following is the best initial treatment option for this patient?

   A. Atropine
   B. Glucagon
   C. Fomepizole
   D. Physostigmine

- **The correct answer is option A.**
- This patient presents with vomiting and diarrhea.
- The physical exam shows miosis, excessive salivation, and bilateral wheezing.
- Vitals signs reveal bradycardia.
- Signs of hypersecretion, along with bronchospasm and bradycardia, suggest an increased acetylcholine activity.
- This morning, the patient took twice the dose of her myasthenia gravis medication due to excessive weakness. Myasthenia gravis is treated with pyridostigmine, an acetylcholinesterase inhibitor. Therefore, this patient has an acetylcholinesterase inhibitor poisoning.
- The best initial treatment option for acetylcholinesterase inhibitor poisoning is atropine. Atropine reverses the acetylcholine effects at the muscarinic receptors.
- Option B is incorrect because glucagon is typically used for the treatment of beta-blocker overdose, not acetylcholinesterase inhibitor poisoning.
- Option C is incorrect because fomepizole is used for the treatment of methanol and ethylene glycol poisoning. Although this patient has a past history of methanol and ethylene glycol poisoning, she has no physical signs or laboratory derangements suggesting these conditions now.
- Option D is incorrect because physostigmine treats anticholinergic toxicity. It does so by increasing the acetylcholine levels in the synaptic clefts. Therefore, giving physostigmine to this patient would further worsen her symptoms.

Emergency Medicine | Section 10: Methanol Poisoning & Ethylene Glycol Poisoning

I. Methanol Poisoning: Definition
  A. Ingesting excessive amounts of methanol

II. Methanol Poisoning: Pathophysiology
  A. Upon ingestion, methanol produces toxic metabolites that lead to symptoms
  B. Metabolized by the same enzymes as ethanol
    1. Alcohol dehydrogenase
    2. Aldehyde dehydrogenase
  C. Methanol is metabolized to formic acid
  D. Causes a high anion gap metabolic acidosis

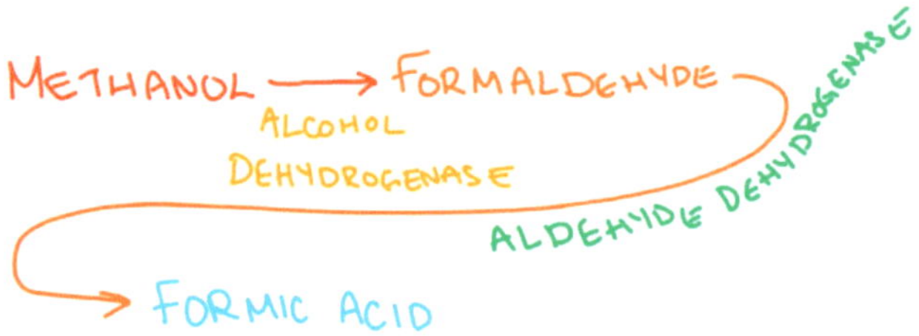

FIGURE 14.1.49 - Methanol Metabolism

III. Methanol Poisoning: Etiologies
  A. Common sources of methanol
    1. Home-brewed alcohol
    2. Antifreeze
    3. Windshield wiper fluid

IV. Methanol Poisoning: Clinical Features
  A. Classic presentation: Anion gap metabolic acidosis + vision disturbances (e.g. blurry vision, central scotoma, blindness)
    1. Formic acid is very toxic to the eyes

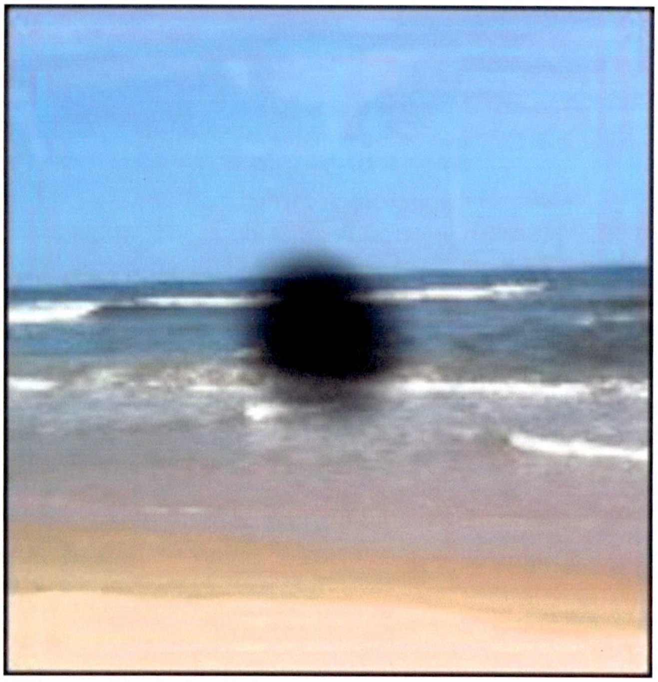

Mick lucas at English Wikipedia, Public domain, via Wikimedia Commons

FIGURE 14.1.50 - Central Scotoma

V. Methanol Poisoning: Diagnosis
  A. Clinical diagnosis
  B. Serum methanol levels (not widely available)
  C. Elevated plasma osmolal gap supports the diagnosis
  D. An elevated osmolal gap narrows the differential diagnoses of high anion gap metabolic acidosis
    1. Ethanol poisoning (rule out with blood alcohol level)
    2. Methanol poisoning
    3. Ethylene glycol poisoning
    4. Other alcohols (e.g. propylene glycol, isopropyl alcohol)

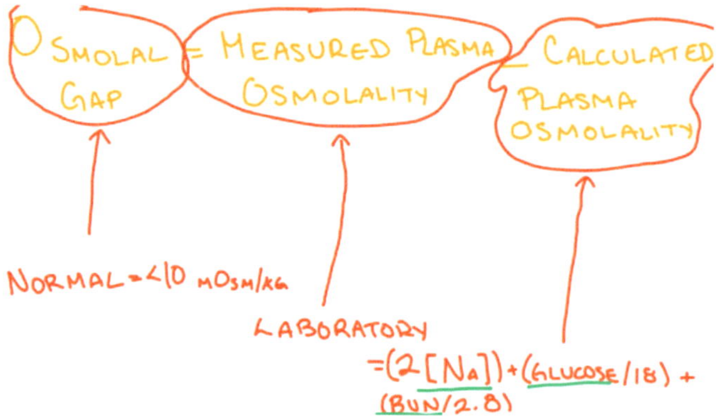

FIGURE 14.1.51 - Osmolal Gap

VI. Methanol Poisoning: Treatment
  A. Supportive treatment (e.g. mechanical ventilation, IV fluids)
    1. Large minute ventilation to correct the acidemia
      a) Patient blows off CO2 → respiratory alkalosis
  B. Fomepizole
    1. Inhibits alcohol dehydrogenase
    2. Prevents toxic metabolite formation
  C. Ethanol
    1. Same mechanism as fomepizole
    2. Can be used if fomepizole is not available

VII. Ethylene Glycol Poisoning: Definition
  A. Poisoning caused by consumption of ethylene glycol

VIII. Ethylene Glycol Poisoning: Pathophysiology
  A. Ethylene glycol becomes converted to toxic metabolites
  B. Metabolized by the same enzymes as ethanol and methanol
    1. Alcohol dehydrogenase
    2. Aldehyde dehydrogenase
  C. Two toxic metabolites of ethylene glycol are glycolate and oxalate
    1. Glycolate and oxalate are acidic
    2. Cause a high anion gap metabolic acidosis
    3. Oxalate also binds to calcium

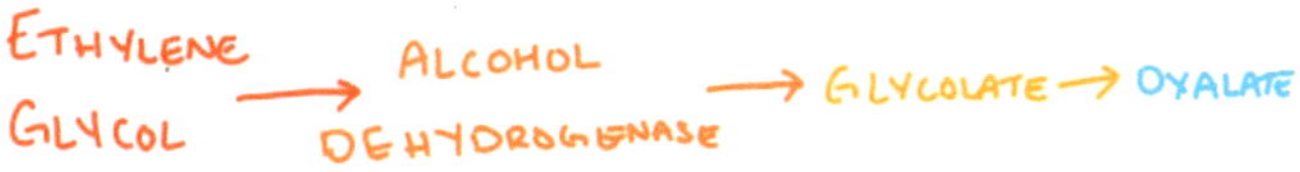

FIGURE 14.1.52 - Metabolism of Ethylene Glycol

IX. Ethylene Glycol Poisoning: Etiologies
   A. Common sources of ethylene glycol
      1. Antifreeze
      2. Windshield wiper fluid
         a. Commonly stored in the garage

X. Ethylene Glycol Poisoning: Clinical Features
   A. Acute renal failure
   B. Calcium oxalate kidney stones
   C. Flank pain, hematuria, oliguria
   D. Hypocalcemia
      1. QTc prolongation
      2. Muscle twitching

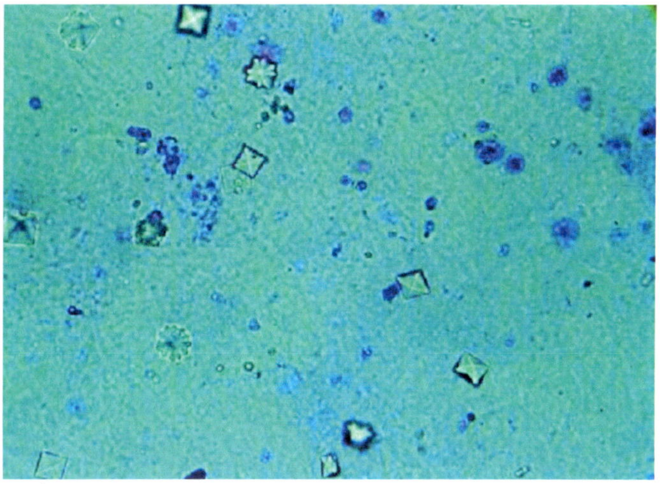

NASA/JSC, Public domain, via Wikimedia Commons

FIGURE 14.1.53 - Calcium Oxalate Crystals

XI. Ethylene Glycol Poisoning: Diagnosis
   A. Clinical diagnosis
   B. Serum ethylene glycol levels (not widely available)
   C. Elevated osmolal gap

XII. Ethylene Glycol Poisoning: Treatment
   A. Fomepizole
   B. Ethanol is an alternative if fomepizole is not accessible

Condition	Etiology	Key Features
Anticholinergic toxicity	- Medications (antihistamines, antipsychotics, TCAs), - Plants (Jimson Weed, Deadly Nightshade)	- "Red as a Beet," " Dry as a Bone," "Hot as a Hare," "Blind as a Bat," "Mad as a Hatter," "Full as a Flask," "Fast as a Fiddle" - No effect on skeletal muscle - Treat with physostigmine
Acetylcholinesterase inhibitor poisoning	- Pesticides containing organophosphates - Physostigmine, neostigmine, edrophonium, donepezil	- CNS depression - "SLUDGE/BBB" - Muscular weakness, fasciculations, paralysis - Treat with atropine followed by pralidoxime
Methanol poisoning	- Home-brewed alcohol - Antifreeze, windshield wiper fluid	- Visual disturbances - High anion gap metabolic acidosis - High plasma osmolal gap - Treat with fomepizole or ethanol
Ethylene glycol poisoning	- Antifreeze, windshield wiper fluid	- Acute renal failure - High anion gap metabolic acidosis - High plasma osmolal gap - Treat with fomepizole or ethanol

TABLE 14.1.9 - Environmental Toxicities

REVIEW QUESTIONS

1. A 3-year-old girl is brought to the emergency department by her parents after accidentally ingesting antifreeze 20 minutes ago. Basic metabolic panel shows Na 139 mmol/L, BUN 14 mg/dl, and glucose 90 mg/dl. The measured plasma osmolality is 308 mOsm/kg H_2O. What is the calculated osmolal gap in this patient?

OSMOLAL GAP = MEASURED PLASMA OSMOLALITY − CALCULATED PLASMA OSMOLALITY

CALCULATED PLASMA OSMOLALITY = 2xNa + BUN/2.8 + GLUCOSE/18

308 mOsm/kg H_2O − 288 mOsm/kg H_2O = 20 mOsm/kg H_2O

- **The osmolal gap in this patient is 20 mOsm/kg H_2O.**
- This 3-year-old girl accidentally ingested antifreeze which contains ethylene glycol.
- Ethylene glycol is a toxic alcohol, the metabolites of which raise the plasma osmolality and result in an osmolal gap.
- Osmolal gap is calculated as the difference between the measured and calculated values of plasma osmolality.
- The measured plasma osmolality is 308 mOsm/kg H_2O.
- Now we need to calculate the plasma osmolality based on serum sodium, bicarbonate, and BUN levels.
- The formula for osmolality is the following: 2xNa + BUN/2.8 + Glucose/18.
- If we plug the numbers in this formula, we receive the osmolality of 288 mOsm/kg H_2O.
- Therefore, the osmolal gap, in this case, is 308 mOsm/kg H_2O - 288 mOsm/kg H_2O.

2. A 47-year-old woman is brought to the emergency department by her partner due to vomiting and severe right flank pain radiating to the groin for the last 2 hours. She has a history of alcohol use disorder. She drank antifreeze when she ran out of alcohol. Laboratory studies are significant for high-anion gap metabolic acidosis. Urinalysis shows envelope-shaped crystals. What is the pathophysiology for nephrolithiasis in this patient?

- **Ethylene glycol ingestion → ↑ oxalate → calcium oxalate crystals → kidney stone.**
- Antifreeze contains ethylene glycol.
- Ethylene glycol is converted into glycolate and oxalate in the body.
- These acids result in a high-anion gap metabolic acidosis.
- Additionally, oxalate combines with calcium in the urine, forming the envelope-shaped calcium oxalate crystals.
- Calcium oxalate crystals then form the kidney stone.
- This is why a patient with ethylene glycol poisoning is predisposed to nephrolithiasis

3. A 37-year-old patient with a history significant for severe alcohol use disorder is brought to the emergency department because of vomiting and confusion for the past 6 hours. Laboratory studies shows:

Na	136 mmol/L
K	3.4 mmol/L
Cl	100 mmol/L
HCO_3-	14 mmol/L
OsM	285 mOsM/kg H_2O
BUN	30 mg/dl
Cr	1.5 mg/dl
Glucose	105 mg/dl
pH	7.29
pCO_2	7 mmHg
pO_2	90 mmHg

The patient complains of blurred vision. Methanol poisoning is suspected, and fomepizole is administered. What is the mechanism of action of fomepizole?

- **Fomepizole inhibits alcohol dehydrogenase and prevents the conversion of methanol into formaldehyde and formic acid. Formic acid is the toxic metabolite responsible for optic nerve injury.**
- This patient presents with vomiting, confusion, and blurred vision.
- Laboratory studies are significant for acute kidney injury, evidenced by high BUN and creatinine. Studies also reveal metabolic acidosis evidenced by low bicarbonate, low pH, and low pCO_2.
- If we calculate the anion gap we find a gap of 22 indicating a high anion gap metabolic acidosis.
- These are the classic features of methanol poisoning for which fomepizole is administered.

REVIEW QUESTIONS

4. A 27-year-old man is brought to the emergency department by his partner because of severe flank pain radiating to the groin for the past hour. He has a history of poorly controlled major depressive disorder. 5 hours ago he drank antifreeze in an attempt to end his life. Vital signs include a temperature of 96.8° F (36° C), blood pressure of 130/80 mmHg, heart rate of 89 beats/min, and respiratory rate of 22 breaths/min. Physical examination shows pain along the left flank, which radiates to the left groin. Costovertebral angle tenderness is absent. Arterial blood gasses reveal pH 7.2 (7.35 - 7.45), HCO^-_3 15 mEq/L (22 mEq/L - 28 mEq/L), and $PaCO_2$ 25 mmHg (33 mmHg - 45 mmHg). Basic metabolic panel shows BUN 15 mg/dL (7 mg/dL - 18 mg/dL) and creatinine 1 mg/dL (0.6 mg/dL - 1.2 mg/dL). Urine microscopy reveals dumbbell-shaped crystals. Which of the following is the best treatment option for this patient?

   A. Ethanol
   B. Fomepizole
   C. Sodium bicarbonate
   D. Dialysis

- **The correct answer is option B.**
- This patient presents with severe flank pain radiating to the groin for the past hour.
- 5 hours ago he drank antifreeze in an attempt to end his life.
- Antifreeze contains ethylene glycol,therefore he is likely suffering from ethylene glycol poisoning.
- Ethylene glycol is metabolized into glycolic and oxalic acids, causing an anion gap metabolic acidosis.
- This patient's arterial blood gas reveals a low pH of 7.2, low bicarbonate of 15 mEq/L, and low partial pressure of carbon dioxide of 25 mmHg.
- Ethylene glycol poisoning is further confirmed by the presence of dumbbell-shaped calcium oxalate crystals on the urine microscopy.
- Oxalic acid produced by the metabolism of ethylene glycol which combines with calcium leading to calcium oxalate crystals.
- The best treatment option for ethylene glycol poisoning is fomepizole.
- Fomepizole inhibits alcohol dehydrogenase, which decreases the production of glycolic acid and oxalic acid.
- Option A is incorrect because although ethanol can also inhibit alcohol dehydrogenase and decrease the toxic effects of ethylene glycol, it is only used if fomepizole is unavailable.
- Option C is incorrect because although this patient has acidemia with a pH of 7.2, sodium bicarbonate is usually not administered unless the pH is less than 6.9.
- Finally, option D is incorrect because although ethylene glycol causes nephrolithiasis and metabolic acidosis, dialysis is not indicated unless acidosis is severe or there are signs of acute kidney injury.
- This patient has compensated metabolic acidosis, and his BUN and creatinine are normal, suggesting intact kidney function.

Emergency Medicine | Section 11: Drug Ingestions & Antidotes

I. Acetaminophen
  A. Hepatotoxicity
    1. Oxidative injury (buildup of NAPQI)
    2. RUQ Pain
    3. Elevated AST, ALT
  B. Nausea, vomiting
  C. Treatment: N-acetylcysteine (NAC)

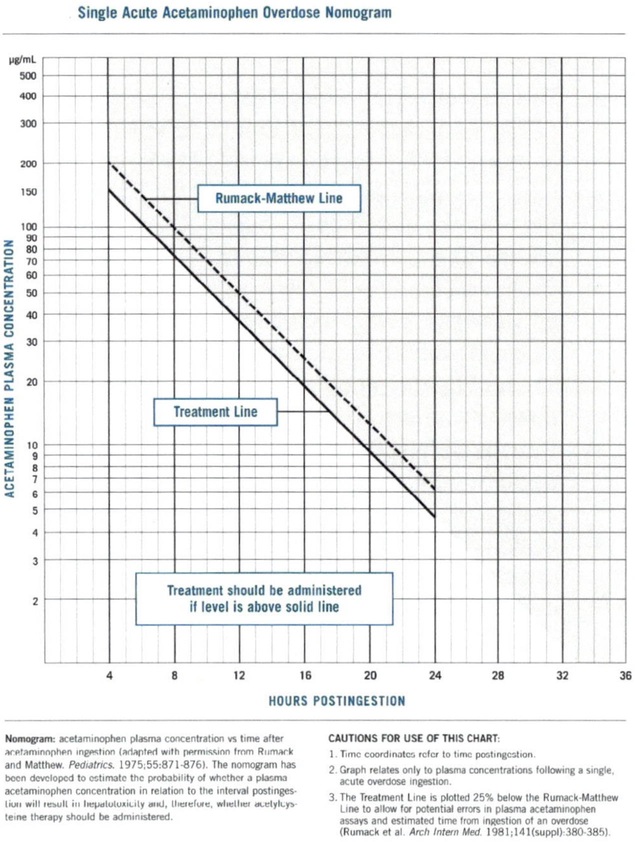

FIGURE 14.1.54 - Rumack-Matthew Nomogram

II. Tricyclic Antidepressants
  A. QT prolongation (Torsades de pointes)
  B. Seizures
  C. Anticholinergic effects
    1. ↑ temperature, flushed skin, dry mouth and skin, mydriasis
    2. Altered mental status
  D. Treatment: sodium bicarbonate (protects against arrhythmia)

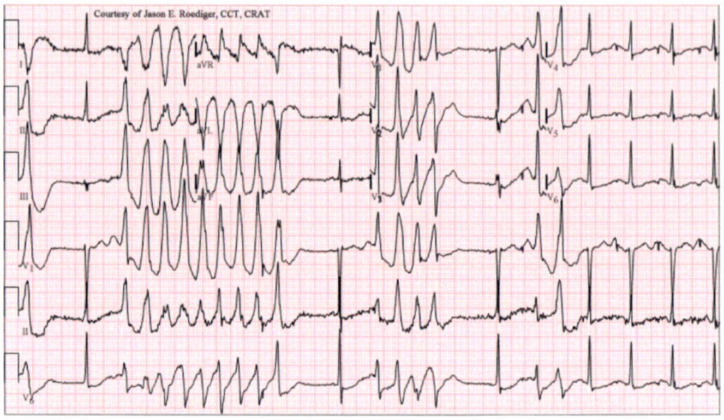

FIGURE 14.1.55 - Torsades de Pointes

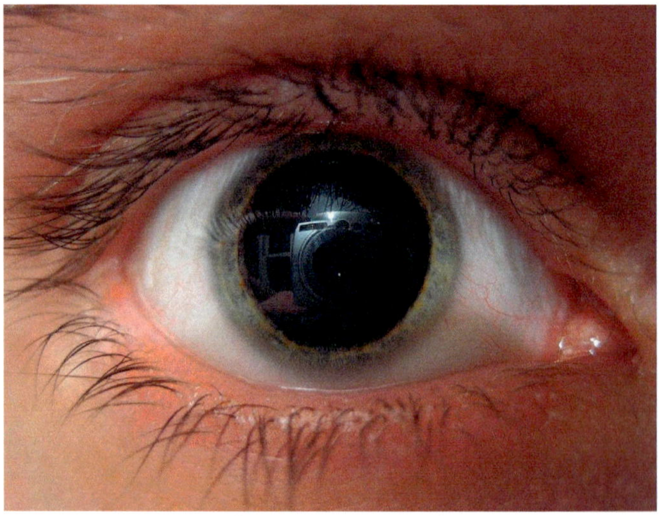

FIGURE 14.1.56 - Mydriasis

III. Opioids
  A. CNS depression
  B. Respiratory depression (life-threatening)
  C. Pupillary constriction (miosis)
  D. Bradycardia
  E. Decreased GI motility
  F. Treatment: Naloxone

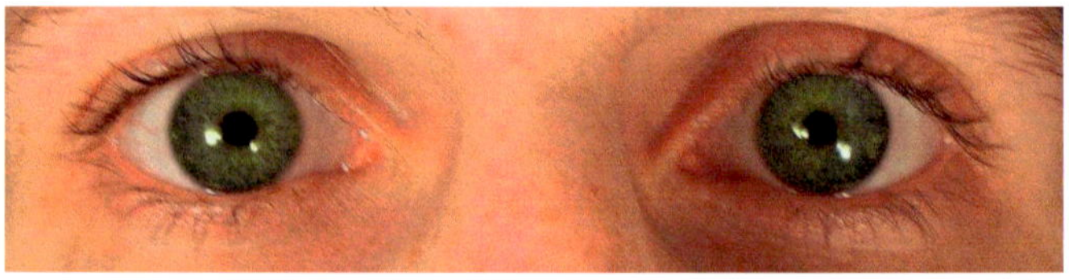

FIGURE 14.1.57 - Miosis

IV. Amphetamines / Cocaine
   A. SNS overactivity
      1. Hypertension, tachycardia, pupillary dilation, fever
      2. Agitation and psychosis
   B. Treatment: benzodiazepines, fluids
      1. If hypertension unresponsive to benzodiazepines, may add
      2. IV antihypertensives, such as nitroprusside or phentolamine
   C. Avoid beta blockers due to unopposed alpha activity
   1. Benzodiazepines
      a. CNS depression
         i. Respiratory depression
         ii. Hypotonia, hyporeflexia
      b. Will not cause "pinpoint pupils" as opposed to opioid toxicity
      c. Treatment: supportive +/- flumazenil (can precipitate seizures)
   2. Digoxin
      a. Xanthopsia: yellow-tinted vision with halos
      b. Hypo/hyperkalemia and cardiac arrhythmias
      c. ECG: "scooped" ST segments
      d. Nausea, vomiting, diarrhea
      e. Antidote: Digibind (digoxin-specific antibody)
         i. Indications: hemodynamic instability, end-organ damage, ↑K+
         ii. K+ levels should be monitored closely

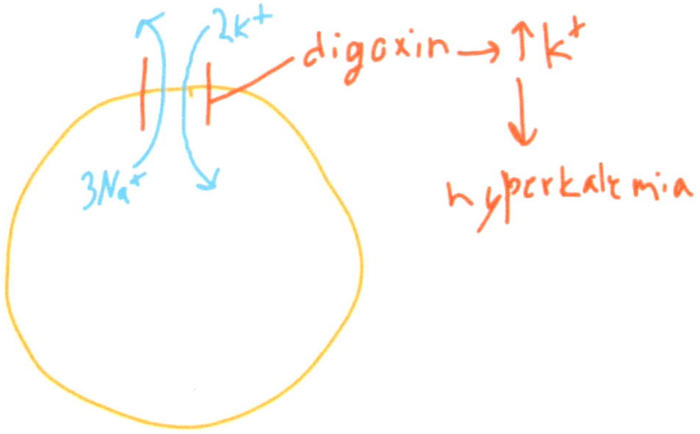

FIGURE 14.1.58 - Hyperkalemia in Digoxin Toxicity

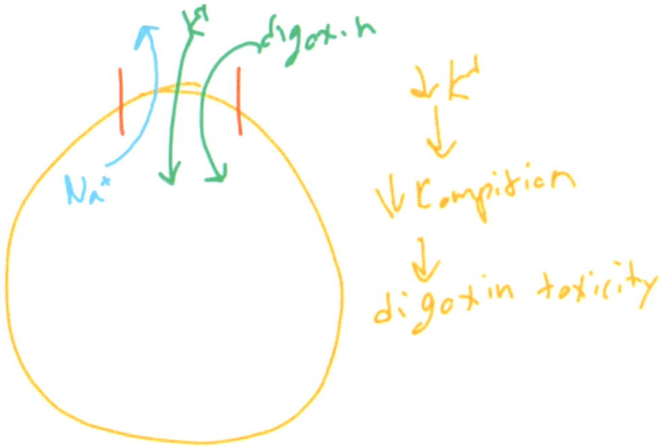

FIGURE 14.1.59 - Hypokalemia in Digoxin Toxicity

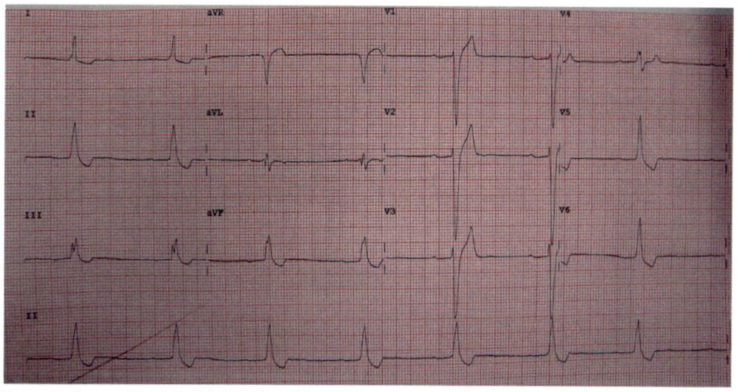

FIGURE 14.1.60 - "Scooped" ST Segments on EKG

V. Anticoagulant Reversal: Heparin
   A. Monitor partial thromboplastin time (PTT)
   B. If life-threatening bleeding, stop heparin
   C. Treatment: protamine sulfate

VI. Anticoagulant Reversal: Warfarin
   A. Monitor PT/INR
      1. INR 2-3: therapeutic level for treatment of atrial fibrillation or thromboembolism
      2. INR > 4: high bleeding risk
   B. If life-threatening bleeding, stop warfarin
   C. Treatment: vitamin K + PCC/FFP

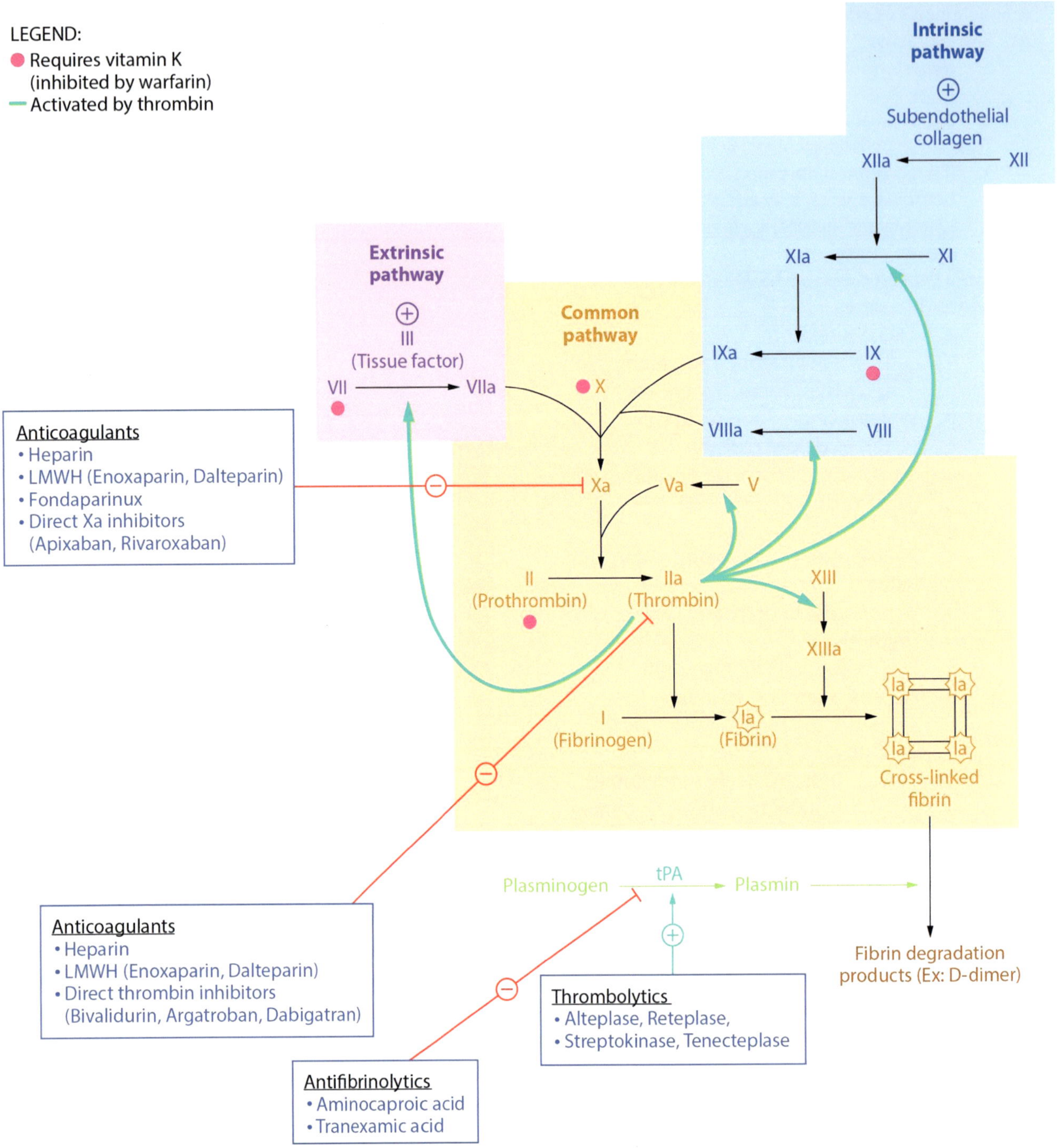

FIGURE 14.1.61 - Coagulation Cascade

VII. tPA
- A. Converts plasminogen to plasmin
- B. Used to treat acute ischemic stroke
- C. If evidence of bleeding, stop tPA
- D. Treatment: aminocaproic acid
  - 1. Inhibitor of plasminogen activators and plasmin

VIII. Beta Blockers
- A. Bradycardia, hypotension, AV block
- B. Bronchospasm
- C. Hypoglycemia
- D. Altered mental status
- E. Treatment: IV fluids, atropine
  - 1. Add glucagon if refractory or profound hypotension

Drug	Toxicity	Treatment/Antidote
Acetaminophen	- Hepatotoxicity	- N-acetylcysteine
Tricyclic antidepressants	- Anticholinergic effects	- Sodium bicarbonate
Opioids	- Respiratory depression - CNS depression	- Naloxone
Amphetamines/cocaine	- SNS overactivity	- Benzodiazepines, fluids (+/- antihypertensives) - Avoid beta blockers
Benzodiazepines	- Respiratory depression	- Flumazenil
Digoxin	- Xanthopsia (yellow vision with halos) - Hypo/Hyperkalemia	- Digibind (anti-digoxin antibody)
Warfarin	- Bleeding	- Vitamin K + FFP/PCC
Heparin	- Bleeding	- Protamine sulfate
tPA	- Bleeding	- Aminocaproic acid
Beta blockers	- Bradycardia, hypoglycemia, hyperkalemia, AMS	- Atropine, glucagon

TABLE 14.1.10 - Drug Ingestions & Antidotes

REVIEW QUESTIONS

1. A 22-year-old male college student is brought to the emergency department by his friends after they noticed him passed out and breathing slowly during a party. He is known to mix his anxiety medication with alcohol, but he seemed particularly "messed up" this time. After initial workup, it is found that this patient has a respiratory rate of 8 breaths/minute, temperature of 37.0C (98.6°F), blood glucose level of 110 mg/dL, and an EKG which shows no abnormalities. What are the next best steps in the management of this patient?

    - **The next best steps for this patient is to offer supportive treatment and monitor this patient's respiratory depression.**
    - This college student has respiratory depression during a party most likely due to combining benzodiazepines and alcohol.
    - Initial workup is normal except for respiratory depression which further backs up the history to confirm benzodiazepines as the most likely ingestion.
    - Flumazenil is the antidote for a benzodiazepine overdose, but it may cause withdrawal symptoms and precipitate a seizure in patients taking benzodiazepines for long periods of time.
    - Since this patient is seemingly prescribed benzodiazepines for anxiety and is known to consistently mix them with alcohol, it is best to administer supportive treatment and carefully monitor this patient's respiratory depression.

2. If a patient who attempted to overdose on acetaminophen 6 hours ago is found to have a plasma acetaminophen concentration of 200 mg/L, would it be recommended to treat with N-acetylcysteine?

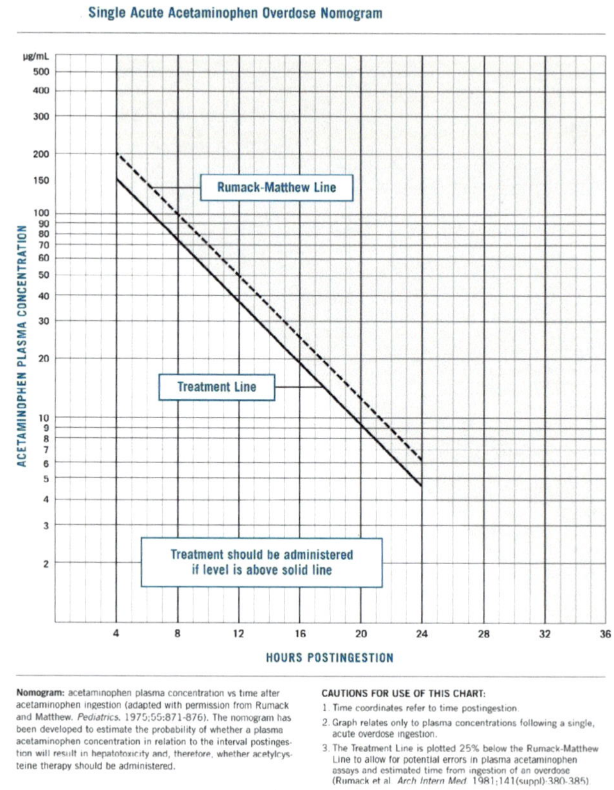

- **This patient should be treated with N-acetylcysteine.**
- This patient ingested acetaminophen 6 hours ago.
- Their current plasma acetaminophen concentration is 200 mg/L.
- Use the Rumack-Matthew nomogram

REVIEW QUESTIONS

3. A 73-year-old man presents to the emergency department after he fell and hit his forearm because it will not stop bleeding. He states that he is taking a "blood thinner" following a knee replacement surgery a few months ago but cannot remember the name of it. Vital signs show a temperature of 37C (98.6°F), heart rate of 112 beats/minute, respiratory rate of 18 breaths/minute, and a blood pressure of 110/70 mmHg. After performing further workup, the patient's PTT is found to be 120 seconds (normal 30-45) and his INR is found to be 1.1 (normal 1-2). Which of the following antidotes should be administered to help stop this patient's bleeding?

    A. Vitamin K
    B. Protamine sulfate
    C. Aminocaproic acid
    D. Prothrombin complex concentrate

- **The correct answer is B.**
- An older man presents due to excessive bleeding after a fall, most likely due to whichever anticoagulant medication he is taking.
- Vital signs are relatively normal other than hypotension, tachycardia which can be attributed to the blood loss.
- After bleeding tests are performed the patient's PTT is found to be 120 seconds which is above the normal limits, and his INR is found to be 1.1 which is normal in healthy individuals.
- Based on this information we can determine that the patient most likely is taking Heparin which would cause an increased PTT.
- If the patient was taking warfarin, we would expect the INR to be increased.
- Therefore, answer choice B is the correct answer because protamine sulfate is the antidote to heparin induced bleeding.
- Answer choices A and D are incorrect because vitamin K and PCC are antidotes for warfarin induced bleeding, and as we mentioned, if this patient was taking warfarin we would expect the INR to be increased.
- Answer choice C is incorrect because aminocaproic acid is the antidote for tPA, a fibrinolytic medication used in the treatment of acute ischemic strokes.

I. Lead Toxicity: Definition
   A. Blood lead level (BLL) of ≥ 5 mcg/dL is considered elevated
   B. Adults
      1. Lead poisoning: BLL ≥ 10 mcg/dL with signs or symptoms
   C. Children
      1. Mild lead poisoning: BLL 5- 44 mcg/dL
      2. Moderate lead poisoning: BLL 45 - 69 mcg/dL
      3. Severe lead poisoning: BLL ≥ 70 mcg/dL

II. Lead Toxicity: Pathophysiology
   A. Absorbed via respiratory tract, gastrointestinal tract, or skin
   B. Deposits extensively throughout the skeletal system
   C. Exerts toxic effects in several ways:
      1. Weakens the immune system
      2. Creates free radicals that damage DNA and cell membranes
      3. Disrupts biochemical pathways by interfering with enzymes (e.g. purine metabolism, vitamin D synthesis, heme synthesis)

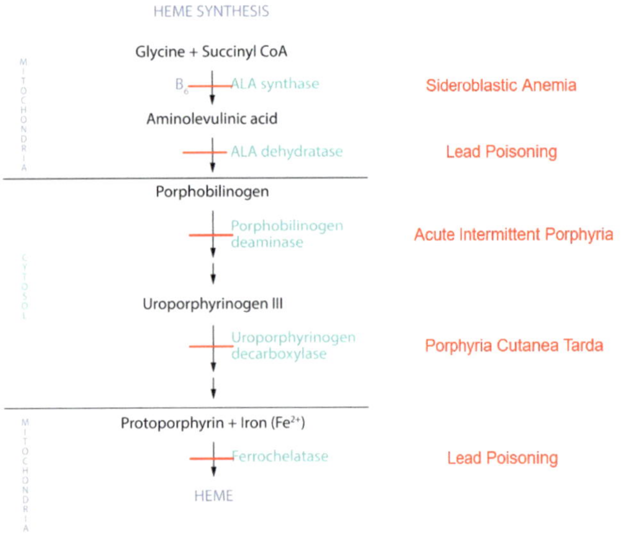

FIGURE 14.1.62 - Heme Synthesis Pathway and Associated Abnormalities

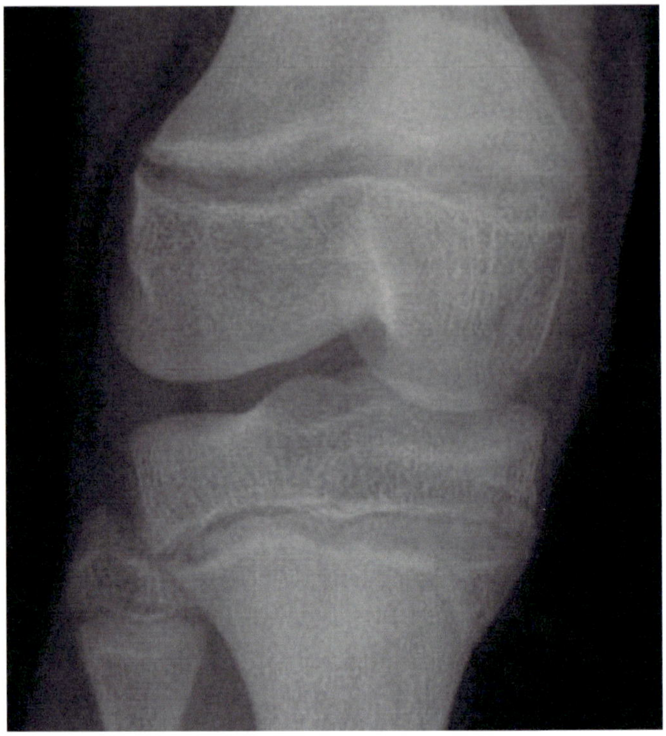

FIGURE 14.1.63 - X-ray of the Knee Joint: Lead Deposition

III. Lead Toxicity: Risk Factors
   A. Adults
      1. Occupational exposure (e.g. plumbing, construction, manufacturing of ammunition or batteries)
      2. Alcohol distillation (parts with lead soldering)
   B. Children
      1. Homes built before 1978
      2. Homes with peeling lead paint or recent renovations
      3. Low socioeconomic status
      4. Recent immigration to the United States
      5. Siblings with known lead poisoning
      6. Pica

IV. Lead Toxicity: Clinical Features
   A. Nonspecific symptoms (e.g. fatigue, irritability)
   B. Gastrointestinal symptoms (e.g. abdominal pain, constipation)
   C. Neurologic symptoms (e.g. neuropathy, cognitive impairment)
   D. Nephropathy, type 2 renal tubular acidosis
   E. Sideroblastic anemia
   F. Burton's line (purple-blue line on gums)
   G. In children, severe lead poisoning (BLL > 70 mcg/dL) can lead to:
      1. Massive cerebral edema
      2. Acute encephalopathy
      3. Irreversible brain damage
      4. Brain herniation

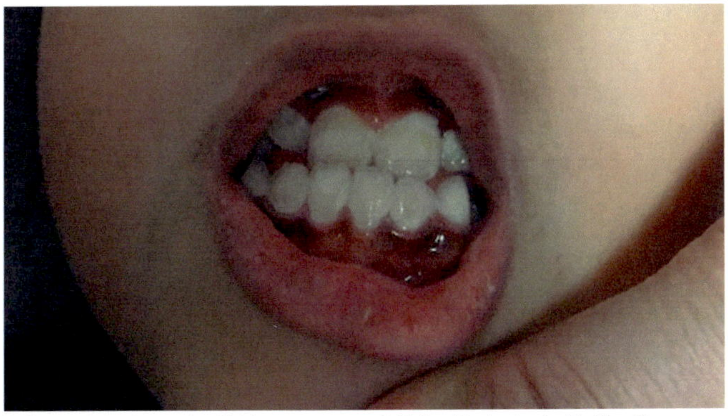

FIGURE 14.1.64 - Burton's Line in Chronic Lead Poisoning

V. Lead Toxicity: Diagnosis
   A. History and physical examination
   B. Labs:
      1. Screening fingerstick lead test for children
      2. Venous lead level
      3. CBC (microcytic anemia)
      4. Serum uric acid (↑)
      5. Serum zinc protoporphyrin levels (↑)
   C. Peripheral blood smear (basophilic stippling)
   D. Bone marrow biopsy (ringed sideroblasts)

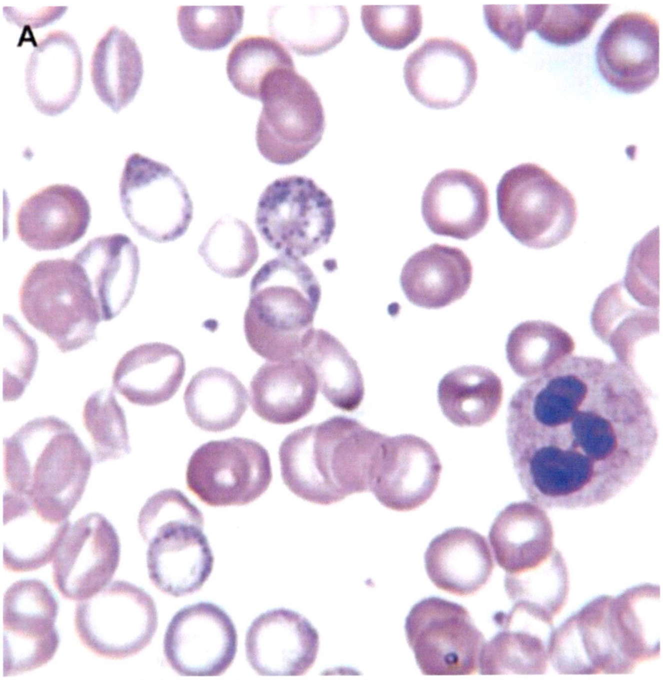

FIGURE 14.1.65 - Peripheral Blood Smear: Basophilic Stippling

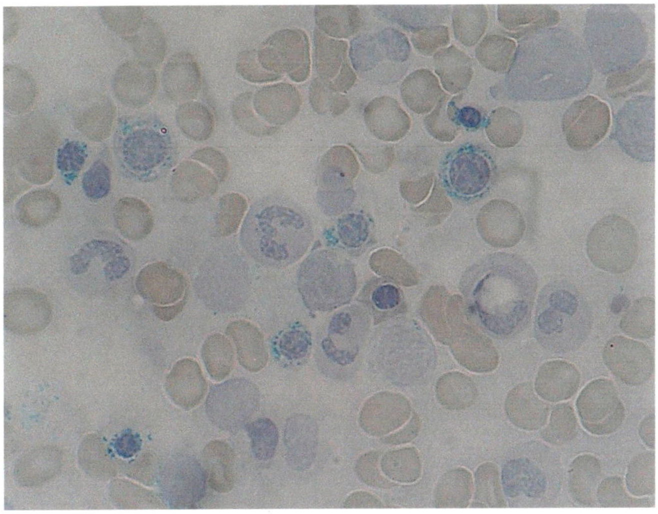

FIGURE 14.1.66 - Peripheral Blood Smear: Ringed Sideroblasts

VI. Lead Toxicity: Treatment in Adults
   A. Eliminate environmental exposure
   B. Chelation therapy
      1. Dimercaprol (a.k.a. British Anti-Lewisite)
      2. EDTA
      3. Succimer (a.k.a. DMSA)
      4. Penicillamine
   C. Activated charcoal is not indicated

VII. Lead Toxicity: Treatment in Children
   A. Children
      1. Mild lead poisoning (BLL 5-44 mcg/dL): eliminate environmental exposure and repeat venous lead level in < 1 month
      2. Moderate lead poisoning (BLL 45-69 mcg/dL): dimercaprol and EDTA
      3. Severe lead poisoning (BLL ≥ 70 mcg/dL): dimercaprol and EDTA

VIII. Arsenic Toxicity: Definition
   A. Exposure to toxic amounts of arsenic

IX. Arsenic Toxicity: Pathophysiology
   A. Tasteless, odorless compound absorbed via inhalation, ingestion, or skin contact
   B. Carried by red blood cells to various tissues and organs
   C. Binds sulfhydryl groups to disrupt enzymes and inhibit:
      1. Cellular respiration
      2. Gluconeogenesis
      3. Glutathione metabolism

X. Arsenic Toxicity: Risk Factors
   A. Soil-derived foods (e.g. rice)
   B. Well water
   C. Pesticides or insecticides
   D. Pressure-treated wood (e.g. outdoor fences)
   E. Arsenic dusts (e.g. smelting, refining, mining)

XI. Arsenic Toxicity: Clinical Features
- A. Acute toxicity
  1. Neurologic symptoms (e.g. encephalopathy, seizures)
  2. Gastrointestinal symptoms (e.g. abdominal pain, watery diarrhea)
  3. QT interval prolongation, torsades de pointes
  4. Garlic breath
- B. Chronic toxicity
  1. Hypopigmentation or hyperpigmentation, hyperkeratosis
  2. Symmetrical sensory polyneuropathy
  3. Pancytopenia
  4. Hepatitis
  5. Mees lines (horizontal white lines on nails)
- C. Latent toxicity
  1. Lung cancer
  2. Bladder cancer
  3. Hepatic angiosarcoma
  4. Basal cell carcinoma
  5. Squamous cell carcinoma

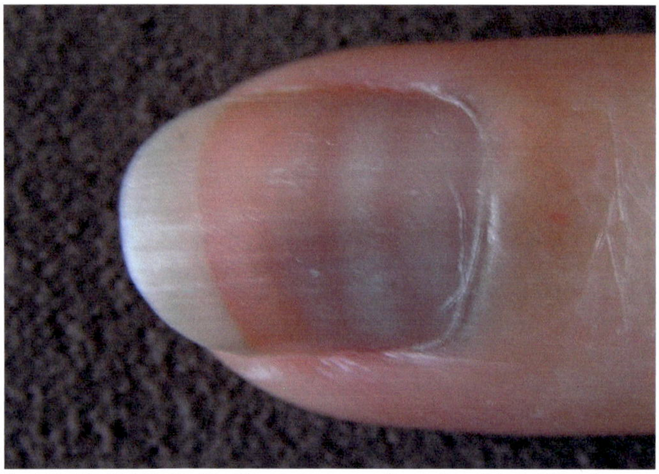

FIGURE 14.1.67 - Mees Lines

XII. Arsenic Toxicity: Diagnosis
- A. History and physical examination
- B. Blood testing is unreliable
- C. Urine arsenic levels
- D. ECG

XIII. Arsenic Toxicity: Treatment
- A. Elimination of environmental exposures
- B. Chelation therapy
  1. Dimercaprol
  2. Succimer
  3. Penicillamine

XIV. Mercury Toxicity: Definition
- A. Exposure to toxic amounts of mercury

XV. Mercury Toxicity: Pathophysiology
- A. Exists in elemental, inorganic, and organic forms
- B. Deposits primarily in the central nervous system
- C. Exerts oxidative damage
- D. Binds sulfhydryl groups to disrupt enzymatic function

XVI. Mercury Toxicity: Risk Factors
- A. Occupational exposure (e.g. felt-processing factories, thermometer manufacturing, mining)
- B. Consumption of fish with high mercury content (e.g. tuna)

XVII. Mercury Toxicity: Clinical Features
- A. Neurologic symptoms (e.g. paresthesias, areflexia, seizures)
- B. "Mad-hatter disease"
  1. Personality changes, ataxia, tremors
- C. Nephropathy (e.g. renal tubular injury)
- D. Lung injury (e.g. interstitial pneumonitis)
- E. Teratogen (microcephaly, cerebral atrophy, blindness, mental delay)

XVIII. Mercury Toxicity: Diagnosis
- A. History and physical examination
- B. Labs:
  1. CBC, CMP
  2. Whole blood mercury level
  3. 24-hour urine mercury level
- C. Chest X-ray in case of significant mercury inhalation

XIX. Mercury Toxicity: Treatment
- A. Elimination of environmental exposures
- B. Chelation therapy using either dimercaprol or succimer
  1. Avoid dimercaprol in cases of methylmercury exposure or extensive central nervous system involvement

XX. Iron Toxicity: Definition
- A. Ingestion of toxic amounts of iron
  1. Unintentional (e.g. children taking pills)
  2. Intentional (e.g. suicide attempts)

XXI. Iron Toxicity: Pathophysiology
- A. Ingested iron causes direct caustic injury to the gastrointestinal tract, which can lead to:
  1. Hypovolemia secondary to fluid and blood loss
  2. Hemorrhagic necrosis
  3. Perforation
  4. Peritonitis
- B. On a cellular level, iron accumulates in mitochondria and leads to:
  1. Disruption of oxidative phosphorylation
  2. Lipid peroxidation
  3. Formation of free radicals
  4. Cell death

XXII. Iron Toxicity: Risk Factors

A. Unsupervised children or improperly stored medicines
B. Young female
C. Suicidal ideation

XXIII. Iron Toxicity: Clinical Features

A. Acute
   1. Gastrointestinal symptoms (e.g. hematemesis, abdominal pain)
   2. Hypovolemia, shock
   3. Anion-gap metabolic acidosis
B. Subacute
   1. Hepatic dysfunction, hepatic necrosis
   2. Renal failure
C. Chronic
   1. Pyloric stenosis or proximal bowel scarring
   2. Symptoms: severe abdominal pain, nausea, vomiting, malaise

XXIV. Iron Toxicity: Diagnosis

A. History and physical examination
B. Labs
   1. CBC, CMP
   2. Serum iron level (peaks 4-6 hours after ingestion)
   3. Anion-gap metabolic acidosis
C. Imaging
   1. Abdominal X-ray may reveal iron in the GI tract (e.g. iron tablets)

XXV. Iron Toxicity: Treatment

A. Airway, breathing, circulation
B. Supportive care (e.g. fluid and electrolyte repletion)
C. Whole bowel irrigation
D. Chelation therapy
   1. Deferoxamine, deferasirox, deferiprone
E. Iron does not adsorb to activated charcoal

Metal Toxicity	Key Feature(s)	Key Management
Lead	- Key risk factors: Adults: occupational exposure Children: homes built before 1978 - Sideroblastic anemia, constipation, neuropathy - Burton's line	- Adults: dimercaprol, EDTA, succimer, penicillamine - Children: treatment depends on blood lead level
Arsenic	- Key risk factors: well water, pesticides, insecticides, pressure-treated wood - QT interval prolongation - Garlic breath - Mees lines	- Dimercaprol, succimer, penicillamine
Mercury	- Key risk factors: occupational exposure, fish with high mercury content - "Mad-hatter disease" - Teratogen	- Dimercaprol, succimer
Iron (ingestion)	- Key risk factors: unsupervised children, suicidal ideation - Anion-gap metabolic acidosis - Pyloric stenosis (chronic manifestation) - Radiopaque iron tablets on X-ray	- Whole bowel irrigation - Chelation therapy: deferoxamine, deferasirox, deferiprone

TABLE 14.1.11 - Metal Toxicity

REVIEW QUESTIONS

1. A 4-year-old girl is brought to the clinic by her mother to establish care. The family recently immigrated to the United States from Sudan. As part of the evaluation, a fingerstick test is performed and reveals elevated lead levels. What is the next best step in management?

    - **The next best step in management is ordering a venous blood lead level.**
    - This child is at risk for lead poisoning due to recent immigration to the United States, which is why a screening fingerstick test was obtained.
    - The next best step in management would be to order a venous blood lead level to confirm elevated blood lead levels and determine the appropriate treatment based on the concentration of lead in the blood.

2. What are the key clinical features that help distinguish lead toxicity from arsenic toxicity?

    - **The key distinguishing clinical features are that lead toxicity can cause nephropathy, type 2 renal tubular acidosis, and Burton's lines.**
    - **Arsenic toxicity can lead to QT interval prolongation, garlic breath, skin changes, thrombocytopenia and leukopenia, hepatitis, and mees lines.**
    - The clinical features of lead and arsenic toxicity in adults are very similar. Both lead and arsenic toxicity can lead to gastrointestinal symptoms, neurologic symptoms, and anemia.

3. A 45-year-old otherwise healthy man comes to see his primary care provider with his wife, who says that he has not been acting like himself lately. He works at an electrochemical plant and attributes his behavior to stress at work and old age. Physical examination shows intention tremor on finger-to-nose testing. When asked to run his right heel down the contralateral shin, the patient was unable to do so smoothly. What is the next best step in management?

    - **The next best step in management is ordering basic labs.**
    - The patient has not been acting like himself lately, which qualifies as a personality change. He exhibited intention tremor on finger-to-nose testing, and he wasn't able to run his heel down the contralateral shin smoothly.
    - Working at an electrochemical plant does increase this patient's risk for mercury toxicity because phenyl mercury can be used as part of the manufacturing process.
    - The next best in management would be to order basic labs, such as a CBC and/or a CMP.
    - A whole blood mercury level or a 24-hour urine mercury level can be ordered to confirm or rule-out exposure to mercury.
    - Similarly, a clinician may also order a venous lead level if there are reasons to suspect lead toxicity, as would be the case if the patient's CBC revealed microcytic anemia, for example.

REVIEW QUESTIONS

4. A 6-year-old girl is brought to the emergency department by her pregnant mother 20 minutes after the girl started vomiting blood. The mother states she noticed a lot of her prenatal vitamins were gone this morning. Initial laboratory evaluation shows anion-gap metabolic acidosis. What findings can be seen on the abdominal X-ray of this patient?

    - **The abdominal X-ray of this patient may show normal findings, radiopaque iron tablets, or air under the diaphragm (perforation).**
    - This child presents with hematemesis and anion-gap metabolic acidosis.
    - This suggests acute iron ingestion on the differential diagnosis.
    - Additionally, this child's mother is pregnant, which means that there are likely prenatal vitamins in the household that the child may have gained access to. Prenatal vitamins have a very high iron content to help prevent iron deficiency in the mother and help ensure sufficient iron supplies for the developing fetus.
    - There are several findings that can be seen on abdominal X-ray following acute iron ingestion.
    - First, the abdominal X-ray may appear normal. Second, it may reveal radiopaque iron tablets. Third, it may reveal air under the diaphragm, which would be consistent with perforation. Perforation of the gastrointestinal mucosa can happen with ingestion of substantial iron quantities due to the caustic injury it exerts on the mucosa.

5. A 49-year-old man is brought to the emergency department from work by his coworker. He says they were working their regular shift at the factory when the patient became confused and lethargic 1 hour ago. Currently, the patient is awake but appears somewhat confused. Review of records from the patient's primary care provider is notable for neuropathy in his feet. The most recent HbA1c was 5.9%. No other conditions are noted in his chart. Vital signs show blood pressure of 134/75 mm Hg, pulse of 98 beats per minute, respiratory rate of 17 breaths per minute, and temperature of 99.0° F (37.2° C). Physical examination shows patchy areas of hypopigmentation and hyperpigmentation on his upper extremities and 1+ patellar reflexes. A stat ECG is ordered and reveals QTc 470 ms. Which of the following laboratory findings would be most consistent with the patient's underlying diagnosis?

    A. Elevated zinc protoporphyrin levels
    B. Pancytopenia
    C. Elevated ferritin levels
    D. Elevated whole blood mercury level

    - **The correct answer is option B.**
    - This factory worker became confused and lethargic at work.
    - His records indicate a history of neuropathy, and a hemoglobin A1c level of 5.9%, which is high enough to call pre-diabetes but not diabetes. Hence, his neuropathy is unlikely to be caused by diabetes and is likely related to toxic metal exposure at work.
    - Physical examination shows patchy areas of hypopigmentation and hyperpigmentation and diminished patellar reflexes.
    - His ECG reveals QT interval prolongation.
    - Therefore, this patient most likely experienced occupational exposure to arsenic and developed pancytopenia as a result.
    - Option A is incorrect because elevated zinc protoporphyrin levels would be expected in a patient with lead poisoning, not arsenic poisoning. Lead inhibits the enzyme ferrochelatase, which is responsible for combining protoporphyrin and heme to form hemoglobin. Inhibition of ferrochelatase will lead to inhibition of heme synthesis and hence build-up of protoporphyrin in the system.
    - Option C is incorrect because elevated ferritin levels would be expected in a patient with iron poisoning, not arsenic poisoning.
    - Option D is incorrect because mercury poisoning is less likely in this patient. Even though the patient does exhibit neurologic symptoms that can be typical of mercury poisoning, his patchy areas of hypo- and hyperpigmentation and his prolonged QT interval are inconsistent with mercury poisoning.

Emergency Medicine | Section 13: Inhalation Injury

I. Inhalation Injury
   A. Nonspecific term for airway irritation
   B. Any part of airway can be affected
   C. Can cause a systemic reaction

II. Inhalation Injury: Pathophysiology
   A. Small particles (< 1μm), heat, or irritants damage the distal airway
   B. Insult to the airway → inflammation → tracheobronchitis and edema
   C. Pulmonary dysfunction and prolonged mechanical ventilation can lead to pneumonia and ARDS

III. Inhalation Injury: Causes
   A. Heat
   B. Smoke
   C. Chemicals

IV. Inhalation Injury: Chemicals
   A. Carbon monoxide (CO)
   B. Cyanide
   C. Arsenic
   D. Ammonia (NH_3)
   E. Mustard gas (agents of war)

V. Inhalation Injury: Smoke
   A. Most often from household or building fires
   B. Can be fatal
   C. Physical exam findings
      1. Burns, singed nasal hairs, soot in pharynx, mucosal ulcerations, airway edema

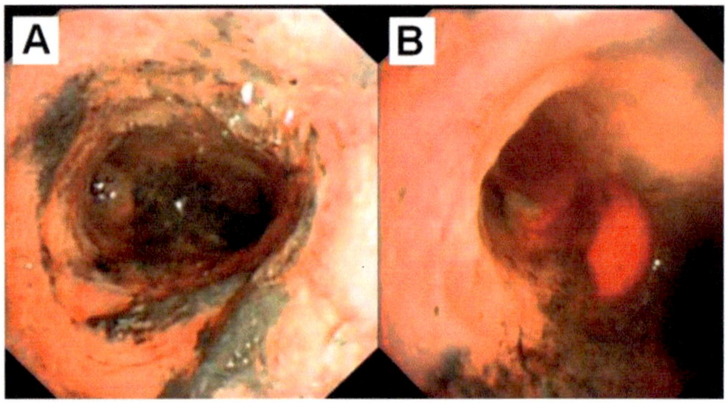

Bai C, et al. 2013. Diagnostic Pathology. doi: 10.1186/1746-1596-8-174

FIGURE 14.1.68 - Bronchoscopy Showing Soot Deposition in the Airway

VI. Inhalation Injury: Treatment
   A. Smoke and heat: supportive care
      1. IV fluids, supplemental O_2, intubation
   B. Chemicals: chemical specific medication

REVIEW QUESTIONS

1. A 25-year-old man is brought to the emergency room by ambulance after being rescued from a burning home 20 minutes ago. He is fatigued and is having difficulty talking in full sentences. He has singed nasal hair and burns on approximately 57% of his total body surface area. IV fluids are started. Shortly after arriving at the hospital he is gasping for air. Physical examination is repeated. Which physical exam finding suggests that the medical team should prepare for intubation?

   A. Singed nasal hairs
   B. Skin burns
   C. Pharyngeal edema
   D. Cherry red skin
   E. Petechiae

- **The correct answer is option C.**
- He is at a high risk factor for inhalation injury because he was rescued from a burning building.
- He has singed nasal hairs and a large amount of burns.
- He is also having difficulty speaking in full sentences, indicating shortness of breath.
- This is concerning for smoke inhalation injury.
- After his IV fluids are started, he becomes increasingly short of breath.
- This is likely secondary to pharyngeal edema from the fluid resuscitation.
- Which would require intubation.
- Option A is incorrect because singed nasal hairs alone do not require intubation, however, they should prompt looking in the patient's mouth at his pharynx.
- Option B is incorrect because skin burns alone do not require intubation.
- Option D is incorrect. However, this might be seen in carbon monoxide or cyanide poisoning.
- Option E is incorrect because petechiae are associated with platelet disorders.

Emergency Medicine | Section 14: Methemoglobinemia and Cyanide Poisoning

I. Methemoglobinemia: Definition
   A. A blood disorder in which hemoglobin is converted to methemoglobin by the process of oxidation
   B. Methemoglobin cannot carry oxygen as well as hemoglobin

II. Methemoglobinemia: Pathophysiology
   A. Exposure of hemoglobin to an oxidizing agent converts ferrous iron (Fe^{2+}) inside hemoglobin into ferric iron (Fe^{3+}), resulting in formation of methemoglobin
   B. Methemoglobinemia produces a leftward shift of the oxygen-hemoglobin dissociation curve, resulting in decreased oxygen delivery to tissues

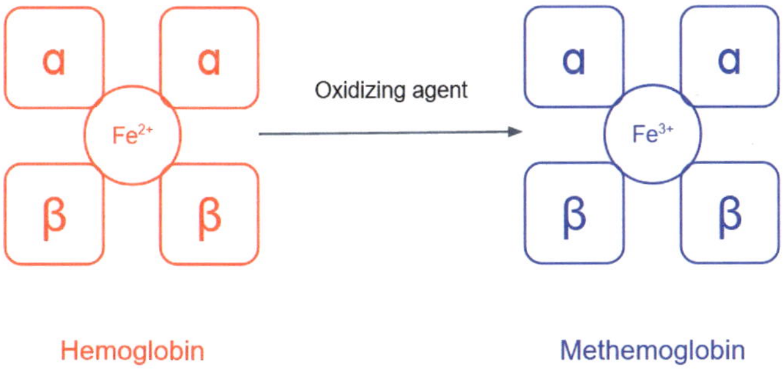

FIGURE 14.1.69 - Hemoglobin and Methemoglobin

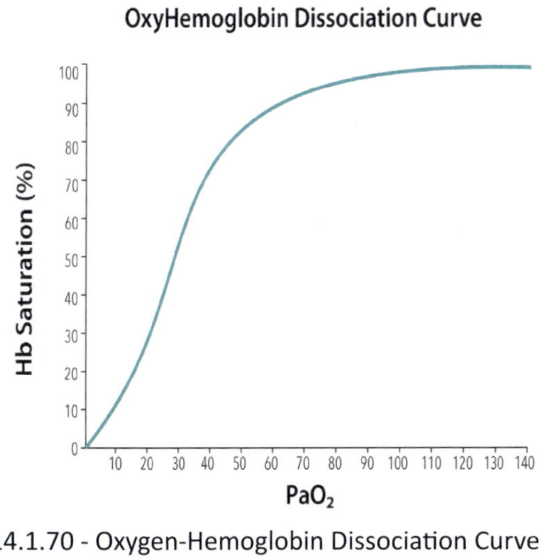

FIGURE 14.1.70 - Oxygen-Hemoglobin Dissociation Curve

III. Methemoglobinemia: Risk Factors
   A. Dapsone
   B. Rasburicase
   C. Silver nitrate
   D. Sulfa drugs (e.g. TMP-SMX)
   E. Local anesthetics (e.g. benzocaine)
   F. Nitrates and nitrites (e.g. drugs, water wells)
   G. Age (infancy)

IV. Methemoglobinemia: Clinical Presentation
   A. Cyanosis
   B. Tachycardia
   C. Respiratory distress
   D. "Chocolate-colored blood"

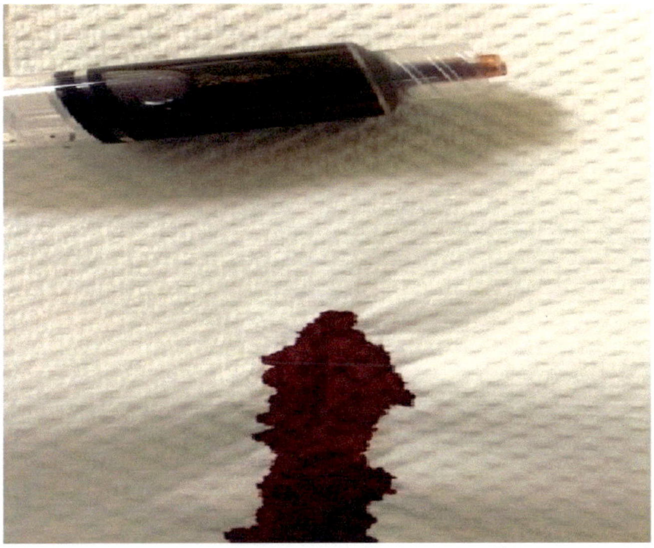

FIGURE 14.1.71 - Chocolate-Colored Blood in Methemoglobinemia

V. Methemoglobinemia: Diagnosis
   A. Pulse oximetry (oxygen saturation will be ~ 85%)
      1. No improvement with oxygen supplementation
   B. Co-oximetry: can measure methemoglobin levels directly
   C. Arterial blood gas (ABG)
      1. Elevated levels of methemoglobin
      2. Normal or high PaO_2, falsely elevated SaO_2
   D. Saturation gap (SaO_2 on ABG - SpO_2 on pulse oximetry ≥ 5%)

VI. Methemoglobinemia: Management
   A. Reduce ferric iron to ferrous iron
      1. IV methylene blue
      2. High-dose vitamin C

VII. Cyanide Poisoning: Definition
   A. Exposure to toxic amounts of cyanide

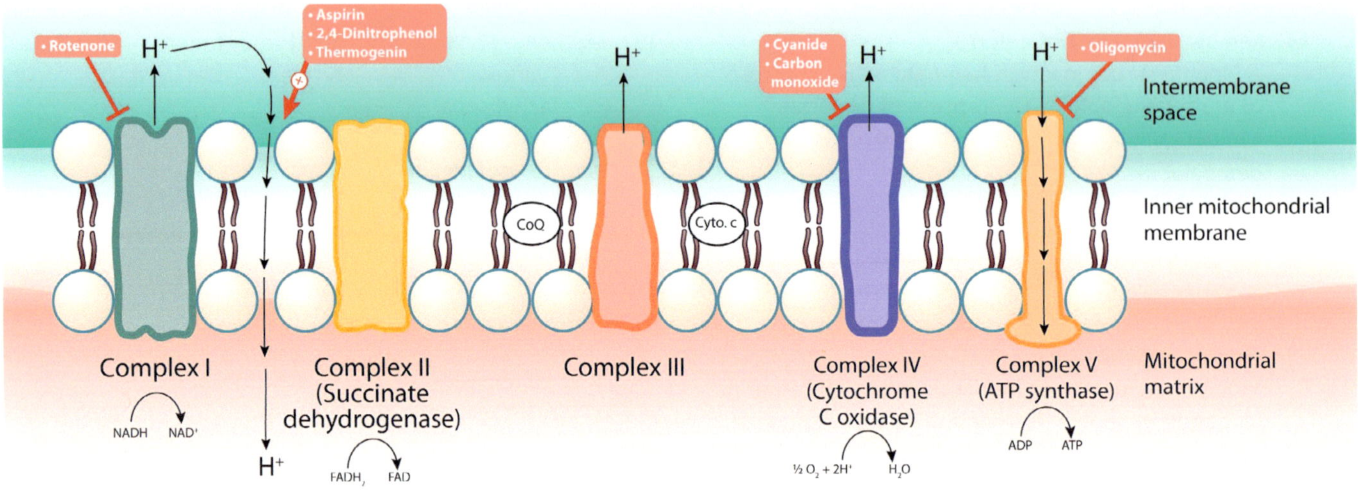

FIGURE 14.1.72 - Electron Transport Chain

VIII. Cyanide Poisoning: Pathophysiology
- A. Cyanide poisoning impairs aerobic metabolism, leading to:
  1. Decreased ATP production
  2. Increased reliance on anaerobic metabolism
  3. Lactic acidosis

IX. Cyanide Poisoning: Risk Factors
- A. Smoke inhalation (especially burning carpets or textiles)
- B. Occupational exposure (e.g. mining, working with pesticides)
- C. Drugs (e.g. sodium nitroprusside)

X. Cyanide Poisoning: Clinical Presentation
- A. Central nervous system: altered mental status, headaches, seizures
- B. Cardiovascular system: tachycardia, hypotension, arrhythmias
- C. Respiratory system: tachypnea, respiratory depression
- D. Renal system: anion-gap metabolic acidosis, renal failure
- E. Gastrointestinal system: abdominal pain, nausea, vomiting
- F. Skin: "cherry-red skin" (early finding), cyanosis (later finding)
- G. Acrid or bitter almond odor on breath

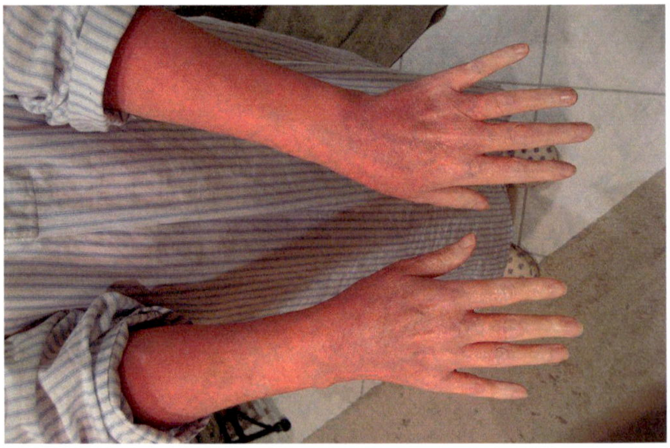

FIGURE 14.1.73 - Cherry-Red Skin

XI. Cyanide Poisoning: Diagnosis
- A. Clinical diagnosis
- B. Serum cyanide test does not result fast enough to be useful for treatment
- C. Lactic acidosis (usually > 10 mEq/L)
- D. Central venous blood gas will show diminished venous-arterial PO_2 gradient
- E. Rule out carbon monoxide poisoning (e.g. carboxyhemoglobin levels)

XII. Cyanide Poisoning: Management
- A. Assess airway, breathing, circulation; perform decontamination
- B. Hydroxocobalamin (first-line)
  1. Binds cyanide to form cyanocobalamin, which is cleared renally
- C. Sodium thiosulfate
  1. Binds cyanide to form thiocyanate, which is cleared renally
- D. Induced methemoglobinemia using nitrites (e.g. amyl nitrate)
  1. Methemoglobin extracts cyanide from cells

REVIEW QUESTIONS

1. Why are infants more susceptible to methemoglobinemia following exposures to various oxidizing agents?
    - **Infants are more susceptible to methemoglobinemia following exposures to various oxidizing agents because of immature cellular pathways, decreased levels of NADH reductase, and increased percentage of fetal hemoglobin.**
    - The cellular pathways responsible for defending against the effects of oxidation are immature or poorly developed during infancy.
    - An example of such a cellular pathway would be the pentose phosphate pathway (PPP), which leads to the production of NADPH - a cellular compound that fuels the antioxidant cellular systems.
    - Infants have lower levels of NADH reductase - an enzyme that can convert methemoglobin back to hemoglobin.
    - Infants have a higher percentage of fetal hemoglobin, which is easier to convert to methemoglobin.

2. A 30-year-old man is brought to the emergency department by his friend in respiratory distress for the last 30 minutes. He is currently being treated with dapsone for dermatitis herpetiformis. Oxygen saturation by routine pulse oximetry is 86%. Arterial blood gas shows a PaO_2 of 95 mmHg and a SaO_2 of 96%. What is the most likely diagnosis?
    - **The most likely diagnosis is methemoglobinemia.**
    - This patient presents with respiratory distress.
    - There is a difference in oxygen saturation reported on pulse oximetry and arterial blood gas.
    - Since this difference is greater than 5%, this patient exhibits a saturation gap, which means the likely diagnosis is methemoglobinemia.
    - In this particular patient, methemoglobinemia was likely drug-induced, as treatment for leprosy often includes dapsone, which has a known association with methemoglobinemia.

3. A 58-year-old man comes to the emergency department with a headache for the past 2 days. Vital signs show blood pressure of 202/125 mmHg. He has end-stage renal disease and is started on sodium nitroprusside. Within the next hour, the patient becomes altered, tachypneic, tachycardic, and experiences a seizure. What is the most likely diagnosis?
    - **The most likely diagnosis is cyanide toxicity.**
    - The patient has received treatment for hypertensive emergency with sodium nitroprusside
    - Sodium nitroprusside poses a risk of causing cyanide poisoning because it is metabolized to cyanide by the body.
    - Usually, the metabolites are cleared by the kidneys. In patients with substantial renal disease, however, cyanide can quickly build up in the system leading to substantial toxicity.

4. How will cyanide poisoning affect the difference in oxygen saturation of arterial blood versus venous blood?
    - **The difference in oxygen saturation will decrease because cells poisoned with cyanide will not be able to extract oxygen from hemoglobin.**
    - Typically, arterial blood rich in oxygen is delivered to tissues where cells extract oxygen, leaving little of it to travel away through the veins and back to the lungs.
    - If cells are poisoned with cyanide, however, tissues will not be able to extract oxygen from the arterial blood, so more oxygen will persist in the venous blood.
    - Hence, if ever presented with venous blood that is rich in oxygen, a clinician should consider the possibility of cyanide poisoning.

REVIEW QUESTIONS

5. A 25-year-old woman is rescued from a burning apartment complex and rushed to the emergency department due to extensive burns on her extremities. She is in severe pain. She has a history of recurrent UTIs, currently treated with prophylactic trimethoprim-sulfamethoxazole. Vital signs indicate Blood pressure of 140/90 mmHg, pulse of 110 beats per minute, respiratory rate of 22 breaths per minute, and oxygen saturation by routine pulse oximetry of 95%. Physical examination shows extensive burns and respiratory distress. She is started on supplemental oxygen, morphine, and local benzocaine is administered to a particularly severe burn on her right lower leg to help control the pain. As the patient is being prepared for the operating room, she suddenly becomes hypotensive, altered, and struggles to breathe despite supplemental oxygen. Which of the following findings would likely be reported on the venous blood gas collected from this patient?

   A. Increased levels of carbaminohemoglobin
   B. Increased oxygen saturation
   C. Decreased oxygen saturation
   D. Elevated levels of methemoglobin

- **The correct answer is option B.**
- This patient presents with extensive burns on extremities.
- She is a victim of a household fire, which means she likely inhaled smoke and was thus exposed to cyanide
- She has tachycardia and tachypnea, and later develops hypotension, altered mental status, and respiratory distress, which is consistent with clinical findings seen in patients with cyanide poisoning
- Exposure to cyanide renders tissues unable to extract oxygen from hemoglobin, which is why oxygen persists on hemoglobin even when it enters venous blood
- Hence, an increased oxygen saturation on venous blood gas is expected, which is why B is the correct answer.
- Option A is incorrect because carbaminohemoglobin is a combination of hemoglobin with carbon dioxide.
- Option C is incorrect because venous oxygen saturation is expected to increase in settings of cyanide poisoning, not decrease
- Option D is incorrect because methemoglobinemia is an unlikely diagnosis for several reasons. First and foremost, the routine pulse oximetry displays a normal oxygen saturation in this patient, while pulse oximeters tend to report a saturation of ~ 85% in patients with methemoglobinemia. Second, methemoglobinemia doesn't usually cause hypotension or altered mental status, although it can certainly cause respiratory distress.

Emergency Medicine | Section 15: Animal Bites

I. Animal Bites: Clinical Presentation
   A. Dog bites
      1. Most common animal bite
      2. May be a crush injury, puncture, or scratch
      3. Adults: extremities
      4. Children: face and neck
   B. Cat bites
      1. Deeper puncture wounds can lead to higher infection rates

II. Animal Bites: Complications
   A. Life-threatening wounds: deep wounds to vital organs can cause major blood loss
   B. Infections: discharge, fever, lymphadenopathy, signs of cellulitis
      1. Pasteurella multocida
      2. *Staphylococcus* or *Streptococcus*
      3. *Bartonella henselae*
      4. Rabies
   C. *Pasteurella multocida*
      1. Common microorganism in dog and cat bites
      2. Gram negative aerobe
      3. Starts as cellulitis but can progress to osteomyelitis
      4. Signs of infection in less than 24 hours
   D. *Staphylococcus* or *Streptococcus*
      1. Gram positive cocci
      2. Both can cause cellulitis
      3. Signs of infection after more than 24 hours
      4. Abscess (*Staphylococcus*)
   E. Bartonella henselae
      1. "Cat scratch disease"
      2. Presents with an initial macule or vesicle in the first week
      3. Progresses to tender regional lymphadenopathy
      4. Immunocompromised: bacillary angiomatosis, osteomyelitis, bacteremia
   F. Rabies
      1. Virus transmitted by the bite of an infected animal
      2. Pathognomonic signs and symptoms: hydrophobia and aerophobia
      3. Additional CNS symptoms: photophobia, seizures, hypersalivation
      4. If untreated, inevitably leads to death
      5. High risk animals: bats, raccoons, skunks, foxes

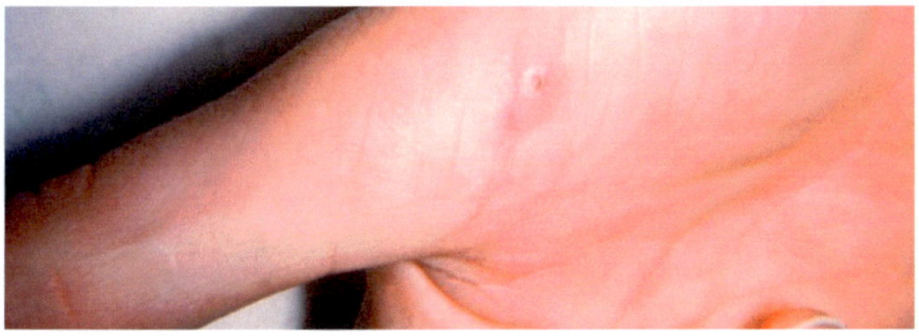

CDC/Public Domain

FIGURE 14.1.74 - Cutaneous Lesion in *Bacillary Angiomatosis*

III. Animal Bites: Diagnosis
   A. Physical exam
      1. Assess hemodynamic stability
      2. Assess the extent of injury, presence of foreign material
      3. Look for signs of infection (fever, tenderness, erythema, drainage)
   B. Laboratory testing: patients with suspected infection
      1. CBC
      2. Blood cultures (aerobic and anaerobic)
   C. Imaging
      1. Deep wounds; near joints
      2. X-ray: fractures, foreign bodies, joint space involvement
      3. MRI: if deeper infections suspected (e.g. osteomyelitis)

IV. Animal Bites: Management
   A. Life-threatening: treat as a major trauma
   B. Non-infected bite
      1. Wound care: stop bleeding, clean, and close the wound
      2. Antibiotic prophylaxis (e.g. immunocompromised, deep wound, proximity to bones or joints)
      3. Simple lacerations can be closed; punctures, cat bites, hand/foot wounds, wounds > 12 hours old should not be closed
   C. Bite that appears clinically infected
      1. Debridement of infected tissue
      2. Wound culture (aerobic and anaerobic)
      3. Blood cultures (immunocompromised)
      4. Antibiotic therapy (e.g. osteomyelitis)
   D. Antibiotic therapy
      1. Infected wounds, closed wounds, deep puncture wounds, and crush injuries
      2. Wounds on hands, face, genitals, or near a joint
      3. Amoxicillin-clavulanate is first line
   E. Determine need for tetanus and rabies prophylaxis
   F. Rabies prophylaxis
      1. Wound cleaning
      2. Active immunization with rabies vaccine
      3. Passive immunization with rabies immunoglobulin

	Clean or Minor Wounds	Dirty or Major Wounds
≥ 3 lifetime doses of tetanus vaccination	- Tdap if last dose of tetanus toxoid-containing vaccine was ≥ 10 years ago - No tetanus immune globulin required	- Tdap if last tetanus toxoid-containing vaccine was ≥ 5 years ago - No tetanus immune globulin required
< 3 tetanus vaccinations, unsure of vaccination status, or unvaccinated	- Tdap - No tetanus immune globulin required	- Tdap - Give tetanus immune globulin

TABLE 14.1.12 - Tetanus Prophylaxis

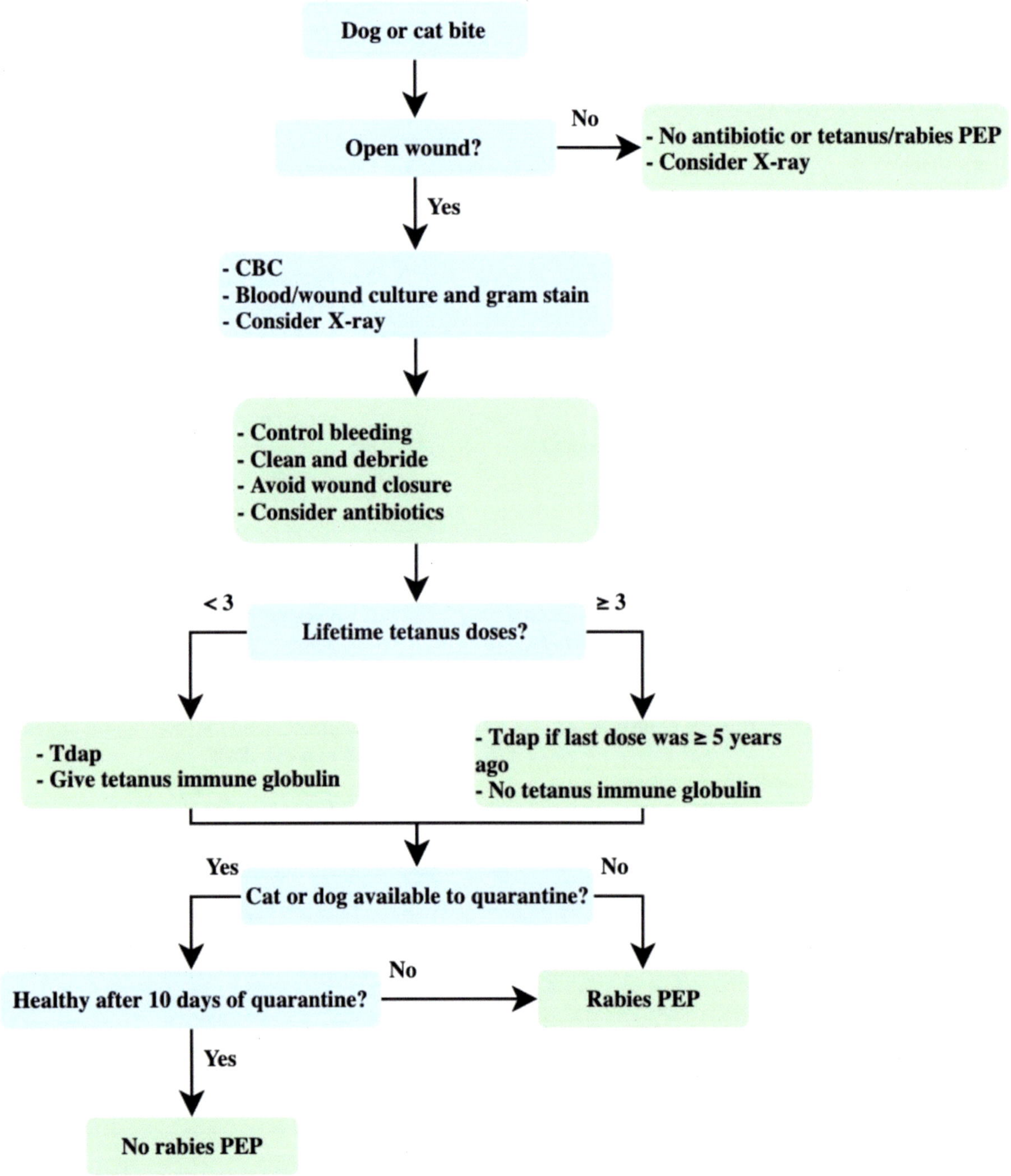

FIGURE 14.1.75 - Rabies and Tetanus Prophylaxis

Condition	Key Features	Treatment
Dog bites	- Cellulitis, rabies, tetanus - Crush or puncture wound	- Antibiotics (amoxicillin/clavulanate), rabies, and tetanus prophylaxis if indicated
Cat bites	- Cat scratch disease; infection - Deep puncture wounds	- Antibiotics (amoxicillin/clavulanate), rabies, and tetanus prophylaxis if indicated
Human bite	- Septic arthritis, osteomyelitis (clenched fist injuries) - Viral infections: HIV or hepatitis	- Antibiotics and tetanus prophylaxis if indicated - Hand surgery for clenched fist injuries
Snake bite	- +/- Envenomation - Coagulopathies, neurotoxicity, cardiac failure	- Stabilize the patient - Antivenin if severe symptoms - Do not tourniquet
Brown recluse bite	- Hemolysis; DIC - Painless bite → red, painful blister → skin and soft tissue necrosis (blue/black)	- Stabilize the patient - Cold compresses to slow necrosis - Debride necrotic tissue - Antibiotics for infection of wound
Black widow bite	- Painful bite → red macule → target-like lesion - Cardiac dysrhythmias, pulmonary edema, muscle spasms and fasciculations, autonomic instability, severe abdominal pain	- Antivenin if severe symptoms - Benzodiazepines for muscle rigidity

TABLE 14.1.13 - Human and Animal Bites

REVIEW QUESTIONS

1. A 35-year-old man comes to the emergency department after being bitten by his neighbor's new dog 1 hour ago. The dog was acting aggressively prior to biting the patient. The neighbor has not had a chance to take the dog in for his vaccinations. What postexposure prophylaxis should be offered to this patient?
    - **The postexposure prophylaxis that should be offered to this patient is cleaning the bite wound, administering the rabies vaccine, and administering rabies immune globulin.**
    - In this scenario, a man is bitten by his neighbor's dog, which is considered a domestic carnivore.
    - Based on the information that the dog has not been vaccinated and that it was acting aggressively, it is of concern that the dog may have rabies.
    - Therefore, it is appropriate to administer post-exposure prophylaxis to this patient.
    - This includes cleaning the bite wound, administering the rabies vaccine, and administering rabies immune globulin to fight the virus during the 7-10 days it takes for the vaccine to stimulate antibody production.
2. A 30-year-old man is brought to the emergency department by his partner after injuring his foot with a rusty axe. Physical examination shows a large dirty wound on his foot. He has had 3 previous tetanus vaccinations, with the most recent being 12 years ago. What is the best next step in management?
    - **The best next step in management is to administer Tdap vaccine.**
    - This patient presents with a large dirty wound, so we are worried about tetanus.
    - He has had three previous tetanus vaccinations.
    - Based on this patient's presentation and that their most recent tetanus vaccine was five or more years ago, the Tdap vaccine would be administered, but tetanus immune globulin would not need to be administered.
3. A 26-year-old man comes to the emergency department after being bitten by a stray dog on the street that he was trying to catch. The dog ran away and has not been located since. The wound is on his calf and does not appear infected at this time. He had limited medical care throughout his life and is unsure of any past medical conditions or vaccinations. After thoroughly cleaning the wound, what postexposure prophylaxis should be given to this patient?

    A. Rabies vaccine, rabies immunoglobulin, and Tdap
    B. Tdap and tetanus immunoglobulin
    C. Rabies vaccine, rabies immunoglobulin, Tdap, and tetanus immunoglobulin
    D. Rabies vaccine and rabies immunoglobulin

    - **The correct answer is option C.**
    - This younger male was bitten by a stray dog whose rabies status is unknown, and the dog is not around for observation.
    - The bite wound is not infected at this time.
    - This patient's vaccination status is unknown, but we assume it to be minimal since he has had limited medical care throughout his life.
    - Therefore, it can be assumed that he has not had three doses of tetanus vaccination, and he will need both tetanus and tetanus immunoglobulin.
    - Since the patient has been bitten by a stray dog, it will be considered a dirty wound.
    - Rabies prophylaxis must be determined.
    - The stray dog ran away, so the animal was unavailable for quarantine.
    - Therefore, the patient will need rabies postexposure prophylaxis.
    - He will need the rabies vaccine and rabies immunoglobulin.
    - Option A is incorrect because it does not include the tetanus immunoglobulin, which is necessary since this patient has a dirty wound.
    - Option B is incorrect because it does not include any post-exposure prophylaxis for rabies.
    - Option D is incorrect because it does not include any prophylaxis for tetanus.

Emergency Medicine | Section 16: Human Bites

I. Human Bites: Clinical Presentation
   A. Usually due to aggressive acts (e.g. assault, abuse); self-inflicted
   B. Tends to cause a crush injury
   C. Clenched fist injuries
      1. Occurs when punching the mouth of another person with a closed fist
      2. Small wounds over the MCP joints

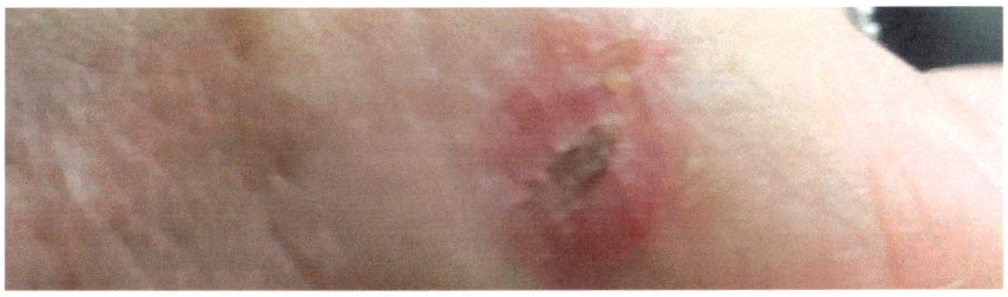

FIGURE 14.1.76 - Clenched Fist Injury

II. Human Bites: Complications
   A. Infections
      1. Mixture of aerobic and anaerobic organisms
      2. Most commonly due to *Staphylococcus* or *Streptococcus*
      3. Rarely may have transmission of viruses
      4. Cellulitis, septic arthritis, osteomyelitis
   B. Fractures or tendon injuries

III. Human Bites: Diagnosis
   A. History and physical exam
      1. Assess location, depth, and nature of the bite
      2. Children: look out for child abuse
   B. CBC: if the wound appears infected
   C. Wound cultures: aerobic and anaerobic
   D. X-ray: concern for fracture or infection close to a joint space

IV. Human Bites: Management
   A. Wound care: stop bleeding and clean
   B. Debride to remove foreign materials
   C. Leave the wound open
   D. Antibiotic prophylaxis for infected wounds, bites on the hands, face, genitals, near joints/ligaments, and crush injuries
      1. First line: amoxicillin/clavulanate
   E. Other interventions:
      1. Determine need for tetanus prophylaxis
      2. Consider testing for HIV
   F. For clenched fist injuries, consider consulting hand surgery

Condition	Key Features	Treatment
Dog bites	- Cellulitis, rabies, tetanus - Crush or puncture wound	- Antibiotics (amoxicillin/clavulanate), rabies, and tetanus prophylaxis if indicated
Cat bites	- Cat scratch disease; infection - Deep puncture wounds	- Antibiotics (amoxicillin/clavulanate), rabies, and tetanus prophylaxis if indicated
Human bite	- Septic arthritis, osteomyelitis (clenched fist injuries) - Viral infections: HIV or hepatitis	- Antibiotics and tetanus prophylaxis if indicated - Hand surgery for clenched fist injuries
Snake bite	- +/- Envenomation - Coagulopathies, neurotoxicity, cardiac failure	- Stabilize the patient - Antivenin if severe symptoms - Do not tourniquet
Brown recluse bite	- Hemolysis; DIC - Painless bite → red, painful blister → skin and soft tissue necrosis (blue/black)	- Stabilize the patient - Cold compresses to slow necrosis - Debride necrotic tissue - Antibiotics for infection of wound
Black widow bite	- Painful bite → red macule → target-like lesion - Cardiac dysrhythmias, pulmonary edema, muscle spasms and fasciculations, autonomic instability, severe abdominal pain	- Antivenin if severe symptoms - Benzodiazepines for muscle rigidity

TABLE 14.1.13 - Human and Animal Bites

REVIEW QUESTIONS

What are the considerations when deciding to treat human bites with antibiotics? What is the first line antibiotic prescribed?

- **It is recommended to treat human bites with antibiotics if the wound is infected; if the bite is on the hands, face, genitals, or near joints and ligaments; and if the bite leads to a crush injury.**
- **The antibiotic of choice when treating human bites is amoxicillin/clavulanate.**

Emergency Medicine | Section 17: Snake Bites

I. Snake Bites: Clinical Presentation
   A. Typically on the extremities
   B. Not all are associated with envenomation
   C. Venomous bites associated with puncture marks
      1. Swelling of the bite site and proximal lymph nodes
      2. Bruising or petechiae near the bite site
   D. Systemic symptoms include dizziness, diaphoresis, nausea, fasciculations

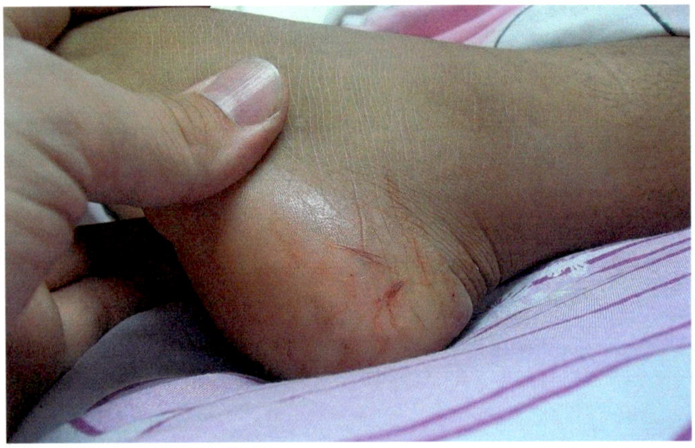

FIGURE 14.1.77 - Puncture Wounds of Snake Bite

II. Snake Bites: Complications
   A. Enzymes in snake venom can lead to:
      1. Coagulopathies and DIC
      2. Increased capillary permeability → distributive shock → hemodynamic instability
      3. Neurotoxicity
      4. Cardiac failure

III. Snake Bites: Diagnosis
   A. Examine the wound and mark the margins
   B. Laboratory testing:
      1. CBC
      2. CMP
      3. Coagulation studies: PT/PTT, fibrinogen, and D-dimer
   C. X-ray: suspicion of a foreign body

IV. Snake Bites: Management
   A. Supportive care to stabilize
   B. Monitor the wound for progression
   C. Analgesia
   D. Antivenin
      1. Side effects: hypersensitivity reactions (anaphylaxis), serum sickness
   E. Tourniquets are not recommended

Condition	Key Features	Treatment
Dog bites	- Cellulitis, rabies, tetanus - Crush or puncture wound	- Antibiotics (amoxicillin/clavulanate), rabies, and tetanus prophylaxis if indicated
Cat bites	- Cat scratch disease; infection - Deep puncture wounds	- Antibiotics (amoxicillin/clavulanate), rabies, and tetanus prophylaxis if indicated
Human bite	- Septic arthritis, osteomyelitis (clenched fist injuries) - Viral infections: HIV or hepatitis	- Antibiotics and tetanus prophylaxis if indicated - Hand surgery for clenched fist injuries
Snake bite	- +/- Envenomation - Coagulopathies, neurotoxicity, cardiac failure	- Stabilize the patient - Antivenin if severe symptoms - Do not tourniquet
Brown recluse bite	- Hemolysis; DIC - Painless bite → red, painful blister → skin and soft tissue necrosis (blue/black)	- Stabilize the patient - Cold compresses to slow necrosis - Debride necrotic tissue - Antibiotics for infection of wound
Black widow bite	- Painful bite → red macule → target-like lesion - Cardiac dysrhythmias, pulmonary edema, muscle spasms and fasciculations, autonomic instability, severe abdominal pain	- Antivenin if severe symptoms - Benzodiazepines for muscle rigidity

TABLE 14.1.13 - Human and Animal Bites

REVIEW QUESTIONS

?

1. A zoo keeper working with snakes was accidentally bitten when he was cleaning the enclosement. This is the first time the keeper has been bitten and quickly received anti-venom. 6-months later this zoo keeper was bitten by another snake and antivenom is given. He quickly becomes short of breath. What is the best next step in management?

- **The best next step in management is to administer an epipen as this patient is having an anaphylactic reaction (type 1 hypersensitivity reaction).**
- It is important to gather information whether they have received antivenom in the past for previous snake bites.
- Anti-venom contains foreign antigens, so after the first exposure antibodies are made in response.
- If the body is exposed to the antigens in the anti-venom for a second time, there is concern for inducing a type 1 hypersensitivity reaction.

Emergency Medicine | Section 18: Spider Bites

I. Brown Recluse Spider Bite: Clinical Presentation
   A. May not remember bite
   B. Painless bite → erythematous border with a purple center → blister → necrosis
   C. Systemic symptoms: fever, malaise, nausea, vomiting, muscle cramps, DIC

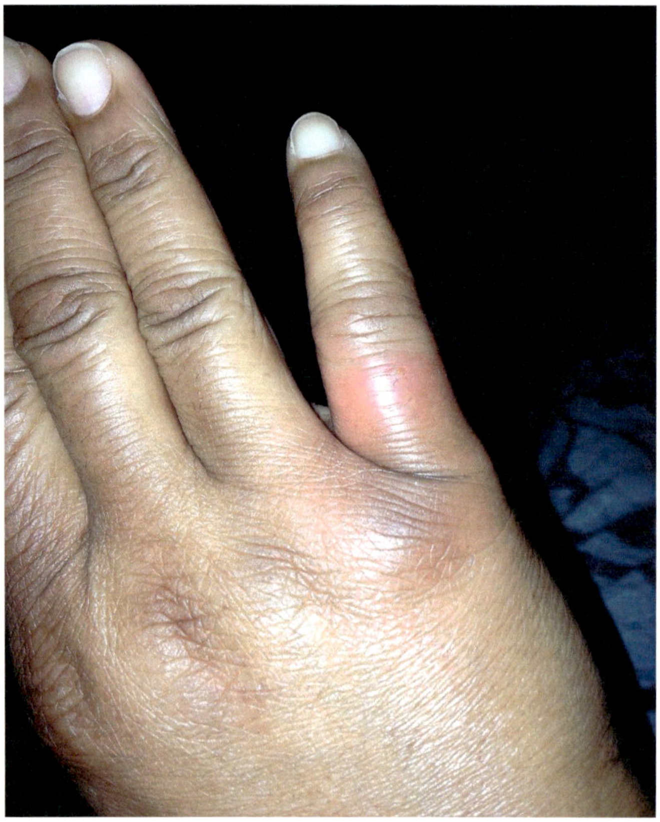

FIGURE 14.1.78 - Brown Recluse Spider Bite

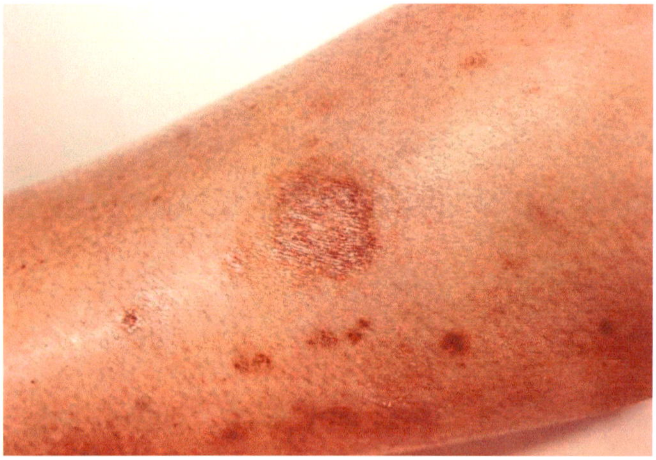

FIGURE 14.1.79 - Scarring After Brown Recluse Spider Bite

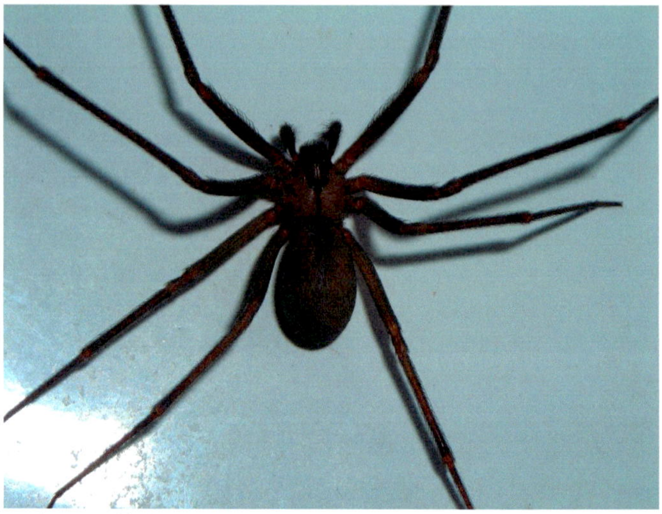

FIGURE 14.1.80 - Brown Recluse Spider

II. Brown Recluse Spider Bite: Complications
   A. Enzymes in brown recluse venom can lead to local tissue destruction
   B. Due to the local tissue destruction, can also have secondary infections in the area of the bite wound

III. Brown Recluse Spider Bite: Diagnosis
   A. Routine laboratory testing and imaging is not required unless systemic signs are present
   B. Labs and imaging: CBC, CMP, PT/PTT, d-dimer, fibrinogen
   C. Consider a plain radiograph of the soft tissue at the bite site

IV. Brown Recluse Spider Bite: Management
   A. Supportive care to stabilize the patient
   B. Clean the wound
   C. Debride necrotic tissue
   D. Antibiotic prophylaxis if infected wound
      1. First line: clindamycin to cover *Staphylococcus*
      2. If severe, consider vancomycin
   E. Tetanus prophylaxis if needed

V. Black Widow Spider Bite: Clinical Presentation
   A. May not remember spider bite
   B. May have burning or sharp pain at the site
   C. Bite site may have two pinpricks from the fangs with swelling and localized diaphoresis
   D. Systemic symptoms: chest pain, palpitations, shortness of breath, headache, cramps, muscle spasms, nausea, vomiting, refractory abdominal pain

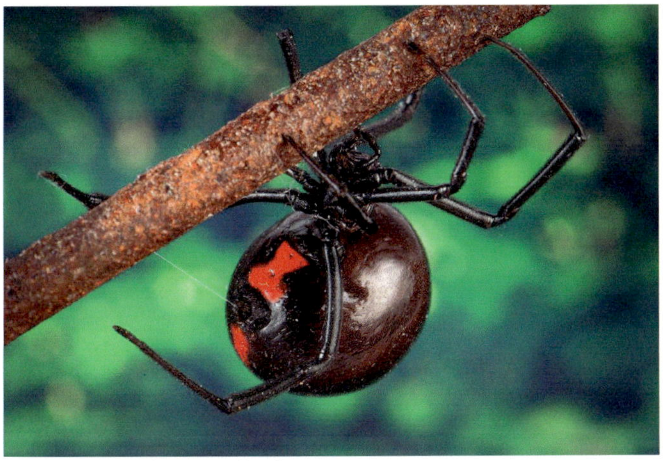

James Gathany, Public domain, via Wikimedia Commons

FIGURE 14.1.81 - Black Widow Spider

VI. Black Widow Spider Bite: Complications
   A. Neurotoxins in black widow venom can lead to:
      1. Cardiac dysrhythmias, myocarditis
      2. Pulmonary edema, respiratory failure
      3. Tetany, fasciculations, tremors, muscle spasms
      4. Autonomic instability
   B. Toxicity secondary to release of neurotransmitters

VII. Black Widow Spider Bite: Diagnosis
   A. No specific tests to detect black widow venom
   B. Laboratory testing:
      1. CBC
      2. CMP
      3. Cardiac enzymes
   C. ECG and cardiac monitoring
   D. Chest X-ray if there are respiratory complaints (e.g. pulmonary edema)

VIII. Black Widow Spider Bite: Management
   A. Supportive care to stabilize the patient
   B. Wound care
   C. Comfort for the patient
      1. Analgesics
      2. Antiemetics
      3. Antihistamines
      4. Benzodiazepines
   D. Antivenin
      1. Severe symptoms
      2. Risks: hypersensitivity and serum sickness reactions
   E. Tetanus prophylaxis

Condition	Key Features	Treatment
Dog bites	- Cellulitis, rabies, tetanus - Crush or puncture wound	- Antibiotics (amoxicillin/clavulanate), rabies, and tetanus prophylaxis if indicated
Cat bites	- Cat scratch disease; infection - Deep puncture wounds	- Antibiotics (amoxicillin/clavulanate), rabies, and tetanus prophylaxis if indicated
Human bite	- Septic arthritis, osteomyelitis (clenched fist injuries) - Viral infections: HIV or hepatitis	- Antibiotics and tetanus prophylaxis if indicated - Hand surgery for clenched fist injuries
Snake bite	- +/- Envenomation - Coagulopathies, neurotoxicity, cardiac failure	- Stabilize the patient - Antivenin if severe symptoms - Do not tourniquet
Brown recluse bite	- Hemolysis; DIC - Painless bite → red, painful blister → skin and soft tissue necrosis (blue/black)	- Stabilize the patient - Cold compresses to slow necrosis - Debride necrotic tissue - Antibiotics for infection of wound
Black widow bite	- Painful bite → red macule → target-like lesion - Cardiac dysrhythmias, pulmonary edema, muscle spasms and fasciculations, autonomic instability, severe abdominal pain	- Antivenin if severe symptoms - Benzodiazepines for muscle rigidity

TABLE 14.1.13 - Human and Animal Bites

REVIEW QUESTIONS

1. A 25-year-old man comes to the emergency department because of chest pain, palpitations, and severe left leg cramping for the past 5-hours. Physical examination shows swelling around the left ankle with two small puncture wounds. What is the most likely offending organism? What can be administered to help ease the discomfort from muscle cramping?

    - **The most likely offending organism is a black widow spider. To help the muscle cramping, benzodiazepines should be administered.**
    - This patient presents with cardiac symptoms of chest pain and palpitations coupled with muscle cramps.
    - The swelling around the patient's ankle with two small puncture wounds suggest that this patient was bitten by an animal, most likely a smaller one like a spider.
    - The swelling and fang marks are more indicative of a black widow spider bite than a brown recluse, which would present as a purple center surrounded by an erythematous border.
    - Additionally, systemic symptoms, such as chest pain, palpitations, and cramping, are more common with black widow spider bites than brown recluse spider bites, which do not typically show cardiac involvement.

Emergency Medicine | Section 19: Immediate & Early Postoperative Fever

I. Postoperative Fever: Definition
   A. Fever > 100.4° F (38° C) after surgical procedure
   B. Self resolves in most cases

II. Postoperative Fever: Pathophysiology
   A. Tissue trauma, inflammation, bacterial toxins
   B. Activation of reticuloendothelial system
   C. IL-1, IL-6, TNF-alpha, IFN-gamma
   D. Preoptic nucleus of the hypothalamus
      1. PGE-2

III. Immediate Postoperative Fever: Etiology
   A. Within a few hours of surgery
      1. Malignant hyperthermia (< 1 hour)
      2. Febrile nonhemolytic transfusion reaction (1-6 hours from a blood transfusion)
      3. Pre-existing infection
      4. Preoperative or intraoperative tissue trauma

IV. Immediate Postoperative Fever: Clinical Features
   A. Malignant hyperthermia
      1. Muscle rigidity, fever, hypercapnia, acidosis
      2. Hyperkalemia, myoglobinuria
      3. Arrhythmia and renal failure
   B. Febrile nonhemolytic transfusion reaction
      1. Fever, chills
      2. Myalgia, nausea

V. Immediate Postoperative Fever: Diagnosis
   A. Malignant hyperthermia (clinically)
      1. Caffeine halothane contracture test, genetic testing
   B. Febrile nonhemolytic transfusion reaction (within 1-6 hours)
      1. Diagnosis of exclusion
   C. Pre-existing infection
      1. CBC, urinalysis, blood cultures
      2. Suspected source of infection (e.g. CXR for pneumonia)

VI. Immediate Postoperative Fever: Treatment
   A. Malignant hyperthermia
      1. Discontinue offending agent, cooling
      2. Dantrolene, high flow 100% oxygen
   B. Febrile nonhemolytic transfusion reaction
      1. Acetaminophen, leukoreduction, termination of transfusion
   C. Pre-existing infection
      1. Antibiotics

VII. Early Postoperative Fever: Etiology
   A. Early postoperative fever: days 0 - 3
   B. Atelectasis (e.g. collapse of a lung, absent gas exchange)
   C. Postoperative pneumonia (e.g. hospital-acquired or ventilator-acquired)
      1. Organisms commonly associated with postoperative pneumonia (e.g. *Pseudomonas*, *Klebsiella*, *Enterobacter*)
   D. Urinary tract infection (e.g. *E. coli*, *Enterococcus*)
   E. Surgical site infection (e.g. group A streptococcus, *Clostridium perfringens*)

VIII. Early Postoperative Fever: Clinical Features
   A. Common in both atelectasis and pneumonia
      1. Tachypnea, dyspnea, cough, hypoxemia
   B. Atelectasis
      1. Decreased breath sounds
   C. Pneumonia
      1. Increased breath sounds
   D. UTI
      1. Urinary urgency
      2. Suprapubic pain, costovertebral angle tenderness
   E. Surgical site infection (SSI)
      1. Pus
      2. Erythema, swelling
      3. Tenderness

IX. Early Postoperative Fever: Diagnosis
   A. Atelectasis or pneumonia
      1. Chest X-ray
         a) Collapsed areas (atelectasis)
         b) Consolidation (pneumonia)
      2. CBC
      3. Sputum and blood cultures
      4. Arterial blood gasses
   B. UTI
      1. Urinalysis (nitrites, leukocyte esterase, pyuria)
      2. Urine culture, CBC, blood culture
      3. Ultrasound
   C. Surgical site infection
      1. Physical examination (wounds, catheters, drain outputs)
      2. CBC, cultures, imaging studies

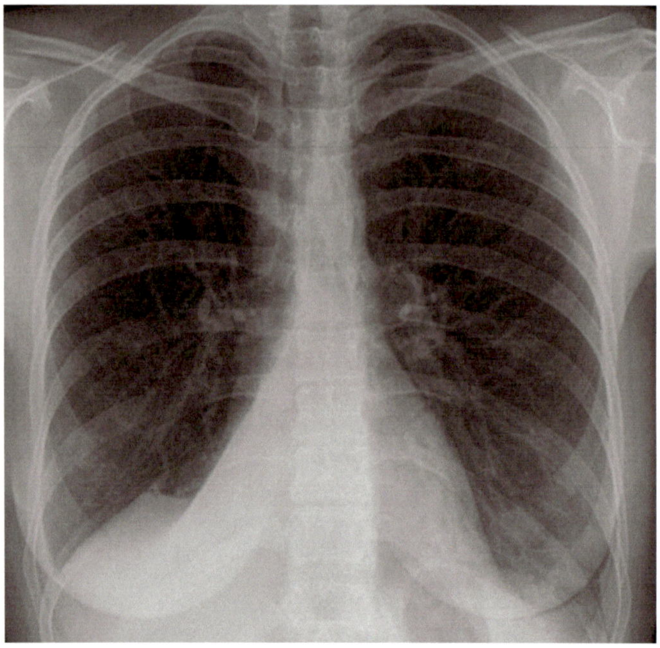

FIGURE 14.1.82 - Chest X-ray: Right Lower Lobe Atelectasis

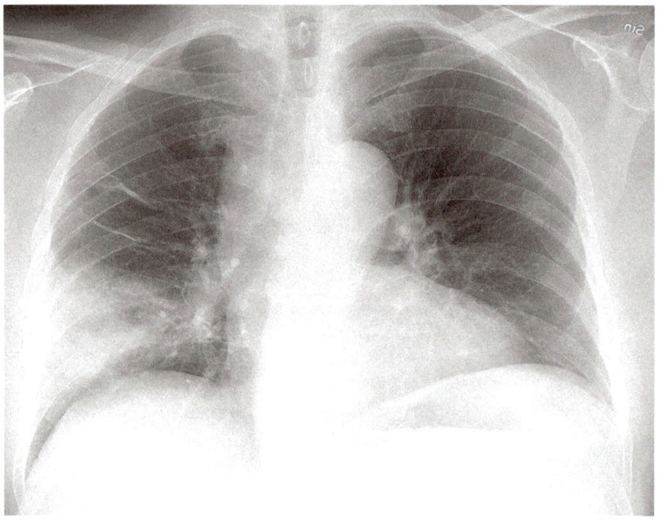

FIGURE 14.1.83 - Chest X-ray: Right Middle Lobe Consolidation

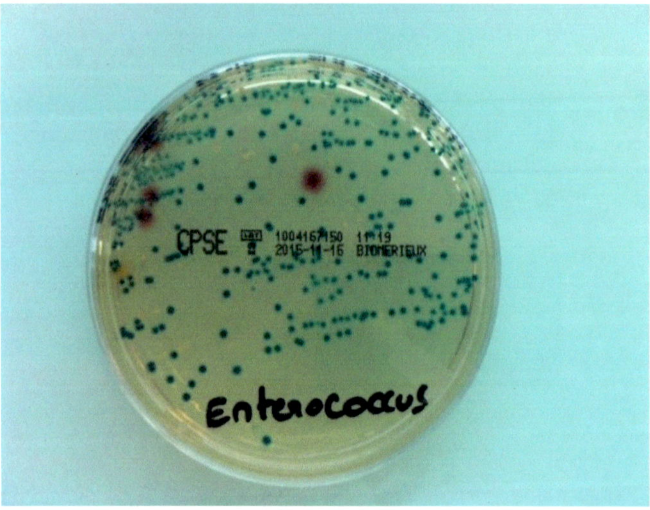

FIGURE 14.1.84 - Colonies of ***Enterococcus*** on Urine Culture

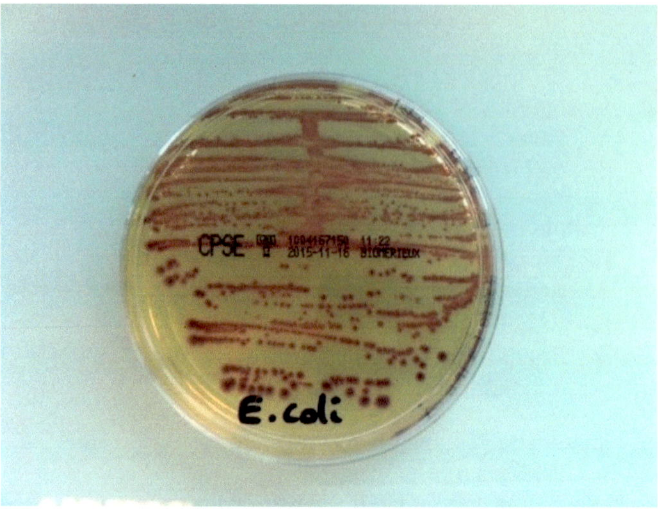

FIGURE 14.1.85 - Colonies of *E. Coli* on Specimen Culture

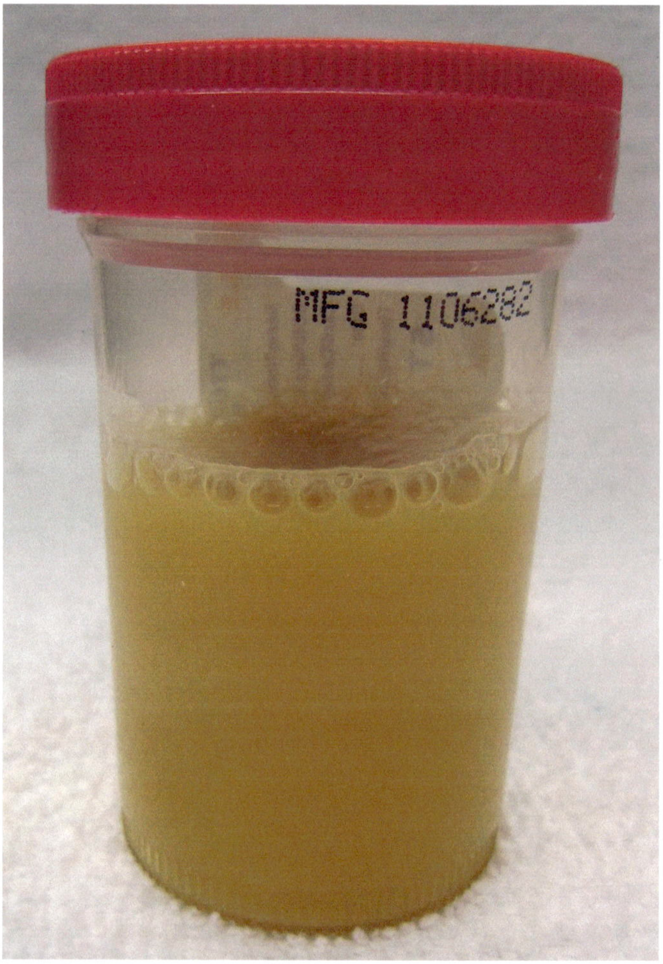

FIGURE 14.1.86 - Pyuria

X. Early Postoperative Fever: Treatment
   A. Atelectasis
      1. Deep inspirations, incentive spirometry
      2. Early mobilization, bronchodilators
      3. Chest physiotherapy
   B. Pneumonia
      1. Oxygen supplementation (SaO_2 < 94%)
      2. Empiric antibiotics (e.g. piperacillin-tazobactam)
   C. UTI
      1. Trimethoprim-sulfamethoxazole
      2. Cephalexin, ceftriaxone
      3. Fosfomycin
   D. Surgical site infections
      1. Superficial: delayed closure, incision & drainage, wound dressings
      2. Deep or severe: antibiotics and debridement

REVIEW QUESTIONS ?

1. A 45-year-old woman was admitted to the hospital and is now on postoperative day 2 following an uncomplicated cholecystectomy. She has now developed a low-grade fever as well as feelings of shortness of breath. Physical examination is notable for diminished breath sounds at both lung bases. The patient is asked to repeat the letter "E" while auscultating both lung bases and "E" is heard clearly. What is most likely the cause for these findings?

- **The most likely cause for these findings is development of bibasilar atelectasis.**
- The patient develops a low-grade fever and shortness of breath on postoperative day 2, which should prompt suspicion for atelectasis or pneumonia.
- Physical examination reveals diminished breath sounds at both lung bases and negative egophony which is more suggestive of atelectasis than pneumonia.
- Pneumonia typically will result in an abnormal egophony test, where the letter "E" is heard to sound like "A", indicating a consolidation.
- A chest X-ray can be ordered to help distinguish between the two likely diagnoses.

2. A 24-year-old G1P1 woman develops a fever and chest pain three days after a complicated cesarean section in which she sustained significant blood loss. She describes her chest pain as sharp and worse when taking deep breaths. Vital signs show blood pressure of 130/75 mm Hg, temperature of 38.6° C (101.5° F), and pulse of 97 beats per minute. Lung examination shows crackles at the right lung base, while abdominal examination shows well-healing incisions without any abdominal tenderness. Pelvic examination is notable for a moderate amount of vaginal discharge that is not malodorous. There is no lower extremity edema or tenderness. Laboratory work-up shows hemoglobin of 9.7 g/dL and leukocyte count of 16,000/mm^3. Which of the following is the most likely diagnosis?

   A. Atelectasis
   B. Pneumonia
   C. Endometritis
   D. Urinary tract infection
   E. Wound infection

- **The correct answer is option B.**
- Three days after a cesarean section, this patient develops a fever and chest pain that appears to be pleuritic in nature.
- Her high fever, pleuritic chest pain, crackles at the right lung base, and significant leukocytosis are strongly suggestive of pneumonia as the most likely diagnosis.
- Option A is incorrect because atelectasis typically results in only a low-grade fever and does not cause such a stark leukocytosis.
- Option C is incorrect because endometritis tends to present with lower abdominal pain and malodorous vaginal discharge. The moderate amount of vaginal discharge described is a normal finding in the immediate postpartum period and is known as lochia.
- Option D is incorrect because the patient was not reporting symptoms suggestive of a urinary tract infection, such as dysuria, and she did not have any suprapubic tenderness on abdominal exam.
- Option E is incorrect because the abdominal exam shows well-healing incisions without any drainage or oozing, making a wound infection less likely.

Emergency Medicine | Section 20: Late & Delayed Postoperative Fever

I. Late Postoperative Fever: Etiology
   A. Days 4 - 30
   B. Deep venous thrombosis
   C. Pulmonary embolism
   D. Drugs (e.g. vancomycin, beta lactams, phenytoin, heparin)
   E. Clostridium difficile
   F. Surgical site infections

II. Late Postoperative Fever: Clinical Features
   A. PE
      1. Sudden shortness of breath, pleuritic chest pain
      2. Tachycardia, hemoptysis
   B. DVT
      1. Sudden throbbing pain in calf
      2. Swelling
      3. Warm, red skin
   C. Drug fever
      1. Nonspecific symptoms (e.g. chills, fatigue)
      2. Diagnosis of exclusion
   D. Clostridium difficile
      1. Abdominal cramps, tenderness
      2. Watery diarrhea
      3. Recent antibiotic use

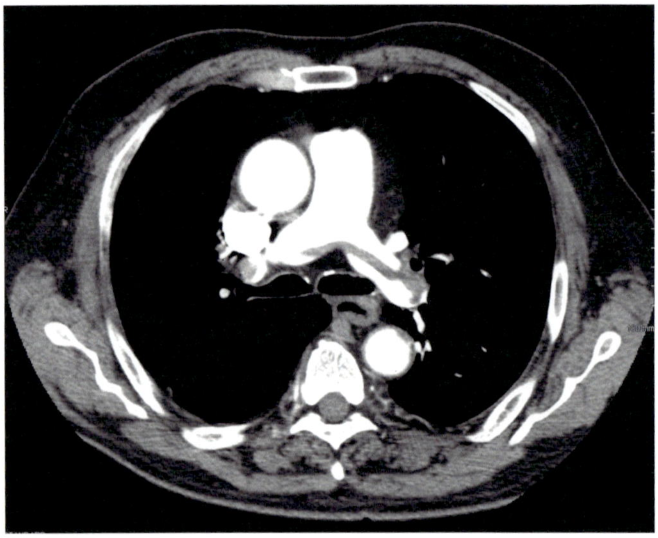

FIGURE 14.1.87 - CT Scan of Chest: Pulmonary Embolism

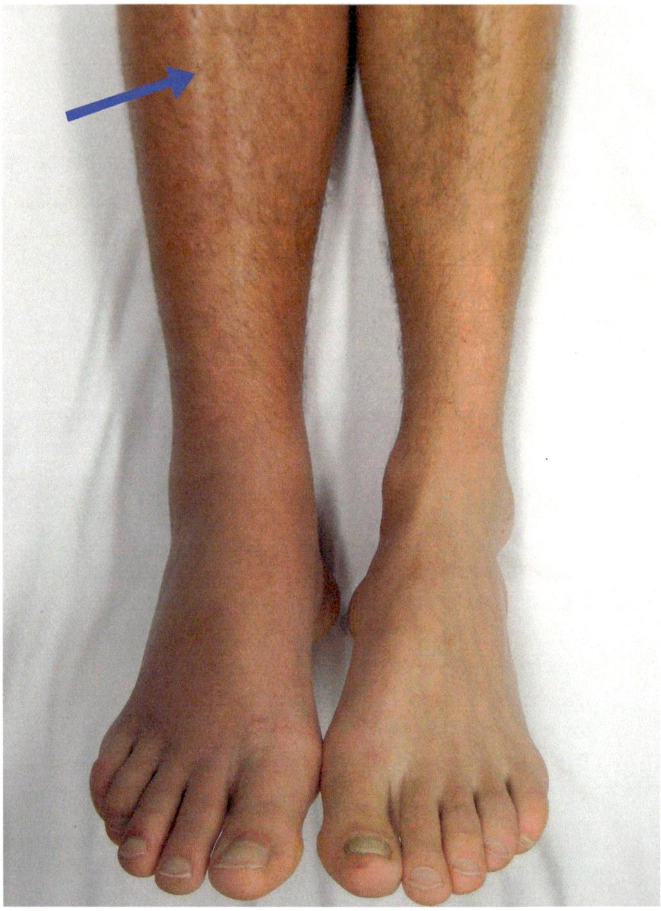

FIGURE 14.1.88 - Red and Swollen Leg in Deep Venous Thrombosis

III. Late Postoperative Fever: Diagnosis
   A. DVT and PE
      1. DVT: Doppler ultrasound
      2. PE: CT angiography (high likelihood), D-dimer (low likelihood)
   B. Clostridium difficile
      1. PCR (detects toxin B)
      2. X-ray or CT (wall thickening or perforation)

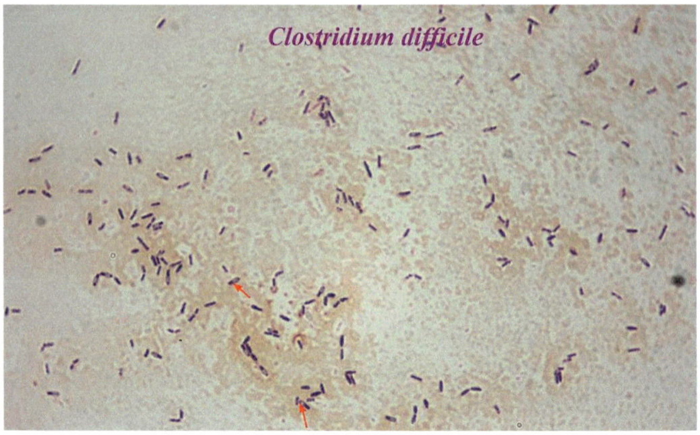

FIGURE 14.1.89 - Gram Stain of C. *Difficile*

IV. Late Postoperative Fever: Treatment
   A. DVT/PE
      1. Heparin
      2. Warfarin
      3. Thrombolysis/thrombectomy (severe)
      4. Inferior vena cava filters (contraindications to anticoagulation)
   B. C. difficile
      1. Discontinue offending medication
      2. Vancomycin
      3. Fidaxomicin
      4. Surgery (severe/refractory)

V. Delayed Postoperative Fever:
   A. > 30 days
      1. Unrelated to the surgery
      2. Infections of implanted devices
      3. Fistula

REVIEW QUESTIONS

1. A 55-year-old woman comes to her primary care physician because of severe watery diarrhea that started 3 days ago. 2-weeks ago she underwent an emergency cholecystectomy for gangrenous cholecystitis. She has been on broad-spectrum antibiotics since the surgery. She has a history of poorly treated type II diabetes mellitus. Vital signs show a temperature of 39° C (102.2° F), blood pressure of 130/80 mmHg, heart rate of 92 beats/min, and respiratory rate of 16 breaths/min. Physical examination shows nontender, nondistended abdomen without guarding and rigidity. Stool PCR for C. difficile toxin B is positive. Which of the following is the best treatment option for this patient?

   A. Erythromycin
   B. Vancomycin
   C. Metronidazole
   D. Exploratory laparotomy

- **The correct answer is option B.**
- This patient presents with watery diarrhea and high fever 2 weeks after cholecystectomy in the setting of recent antibiotic use.
- The timeframe of her fever is consistent with the late postoperative fever.
- She has been on broad-spectrum antibiotic regimen since the surgery.
- Additionally, stool PCR for toxin B is positive.
- All these findings are consistent with the diagnosis of pseudomembranous colitis caused by *C. difficile*.
- The best initial treatment option for uncomplicated pseudomembranous colitis is vancomycin.
- Option A, erythromycin, is incorrect because it is not used in the management of pseudomembranous colitis.
- Option C, metronidazole, is incorrect because it is mostly used in patients with fulminant C. Difficile colitis, characterized by hypotension, tachycardia, and signs of toxic megacolon.
- However, even in fulminant colitis, vancomycin and fidaxomicin are preferred over metronidazole.
- Option D, exploratory laparotomy, is indicated in patients with colonic perforation and peritonitis. This patient has normal abdominal exam findings, without signs of peritonitis or perforation and thus does not need surgical intervention.

TABLES & FIGURES

Made in the USA
Las Vegas, NV
03 November 2026

57423930R00050